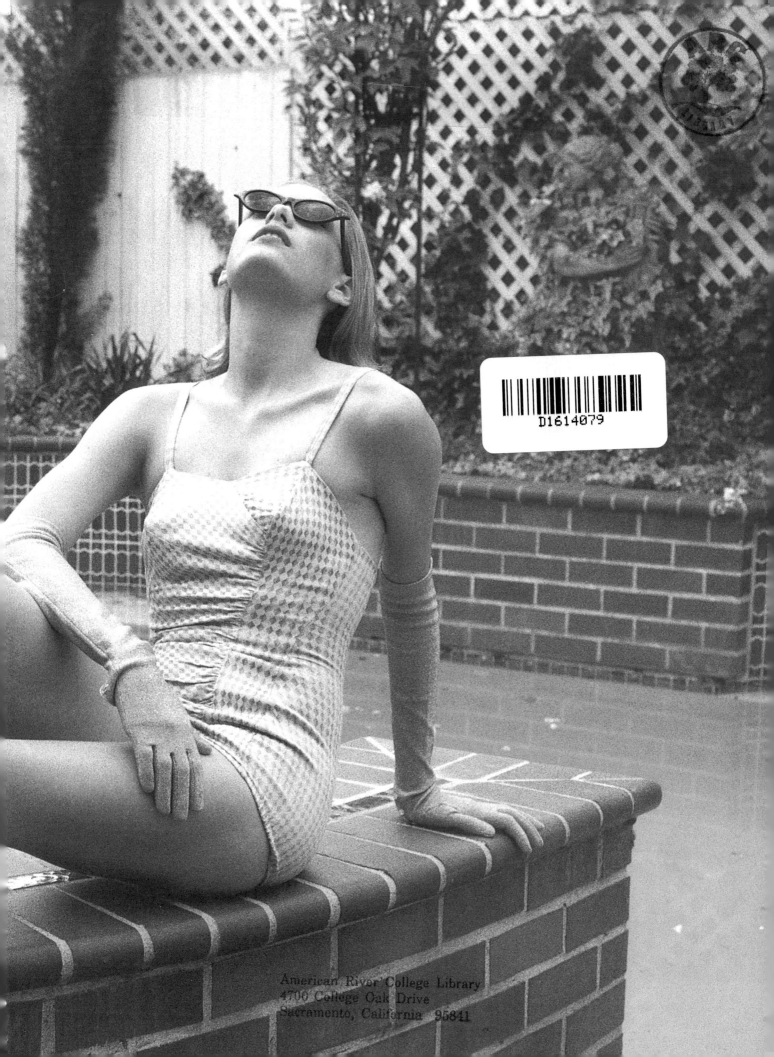

California Casual

FASHIONS, 1930s-1970s

Maureen Reilly

Schiffer Publishing Ltd®

4880 Lower Valley Road, Atglen, PA 19310 USA

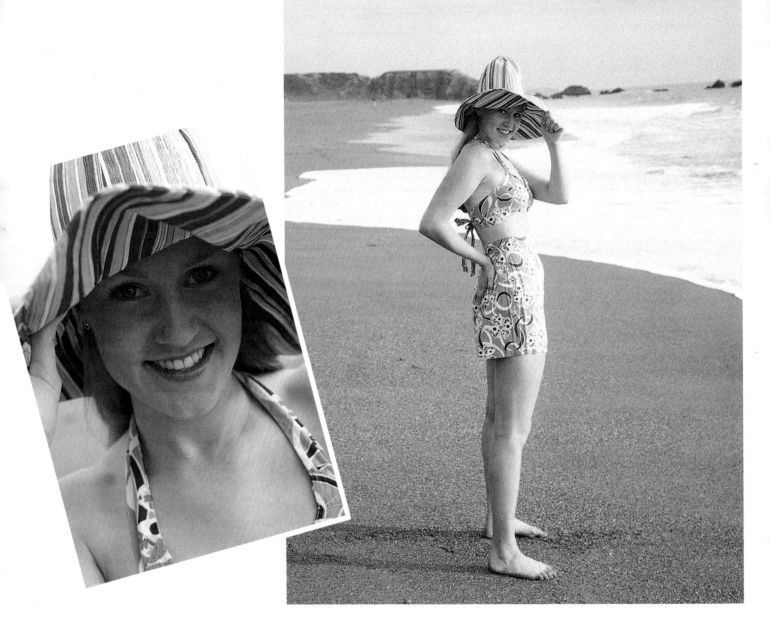

Cover image: Advertisement for Rose Marie Reid swimsuit and jacket, as shown in *Harper's Bazaar*, January, 1961.

Copyright © 2001 by Maureen Reilly
Library of Congress Card Number: 00-111049

Designed by Bonnie M. Hensley
Cover design by Bruce M. Waters
Type set in Aldine 721 BT/ZapfHumanist BT

ISBN: 0-7643-1246-4
Printed in China
1 2 3 4

Published by Schiffer Publishing Ltd.
4880 Lower Valley Road
Atglen, PA 19310
Phone: (610) 593-1777; Fax: (610) 593-2002
E-mail: Schifferbk@aol.com
Please visit our web site catalog at
www.schifferbooks.com

We are always looking for people to write books on new and related subjects. If you have an idea for a book, please contact us at the above address.
This book may be purchased from the publisher.
Include $3.95 for shipping.
Please try your bookstore first.
You may write for a free catalog.

In Europe, Schiffer books are distributed by
Bushwood Books
6 Marksbury Avenue
Kew Gardens
Surrey TW9 4JF England
Phone: 44 (0) 20 8392 8585
Fax: 44 (0) 20 8392 9876
E-mail: Bushwd@aol.com
Free postage in the UK. Europe: air mail at cost.

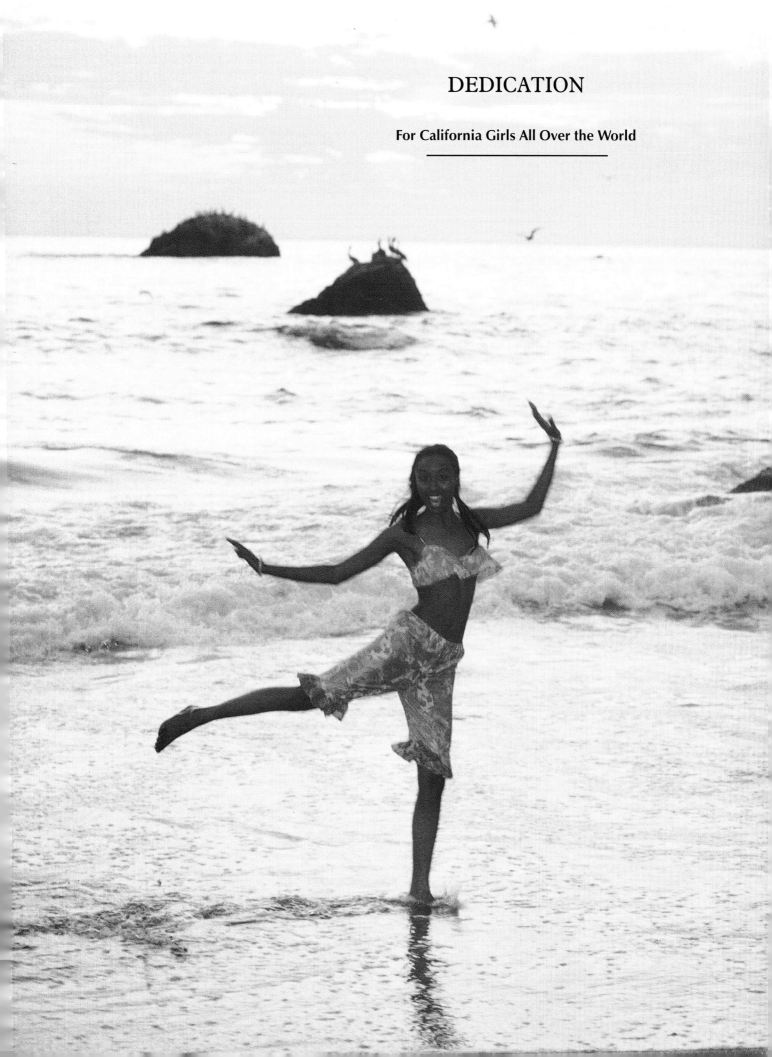

DEDICATION

For California Girls All Over the World

ACKNOWLEDGMENTS

With heartfelt thanks to the many vintage clothing dealers and collectors who graciously loaned garments for the photographs in this book—especially to Marlene Davenport with *Cheap Thrills* in Sacramento, Lis Normoyle with *Luxe* in Palo Alto, and Doris Raymond with *The Way We Wore* in San Francisco.

This book could not have been produced without the wonderful photography of John Klycinski and Gideon Dominguez, nor the assistance of *Just 4 Kids* model and talent agency. Plaudits are also due to the models themselves, who are named throughout the book. A special mention goes to Jimmy Mitchell, who modeled swimsuits and sportswear throughout the 1950s and 1960s, and whose generous release of original photos helped bring this book into focus.

A special acknowledgment is due to JoAnn Stabb, Senior Lecturer and Design Curator for the Design Collection, Department of Environmental Design at the University of California at Davis, for her assistance with my original research. Also, to Anne Cole, who generously loaned vintage ads and photos from her own archives.

Finally, thanks to my editor Donna Baker and the staff at Schiffer Publishing, for all of their help and support in producing a quality book.

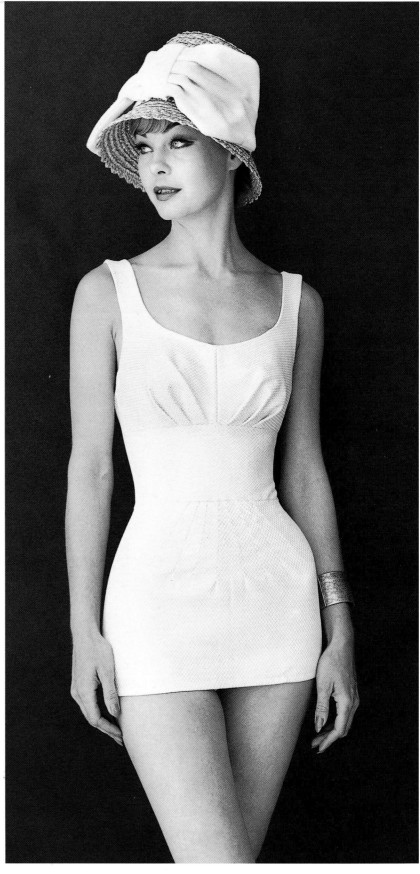

CONTENTS

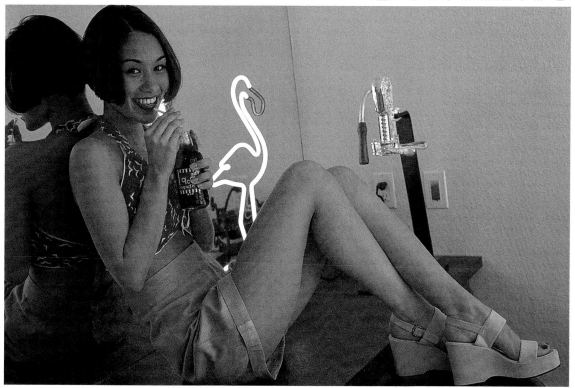

Opposite page
Jimmy Mitchell modeled for Rose Marie Reid in the late 1950s. She also posed for Catalina, Cole, Lanz, and many other California companies, and was the first photography model for award-winning sportswear designer Rudi Gernreich.

INTRODUCTION

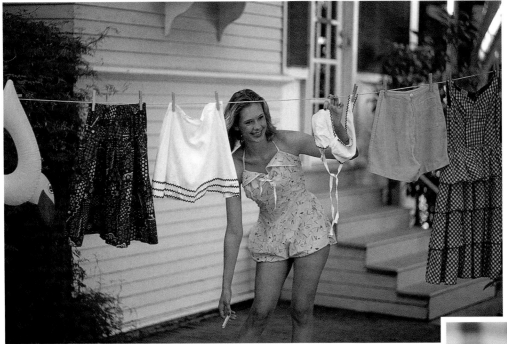

California—a state that joined the union as a hasty postscript to the gold rush of 1849, became a haven for dustbowl immigrants in 1939, and gloried in the glamour of Hollywood from the days of silent films to Cinemax. Blessed with a fertile soil, sunny clime, and miles of coastline—California is not just a state, but a state of mind. Could there be a better birthplace for the sportswear industry?

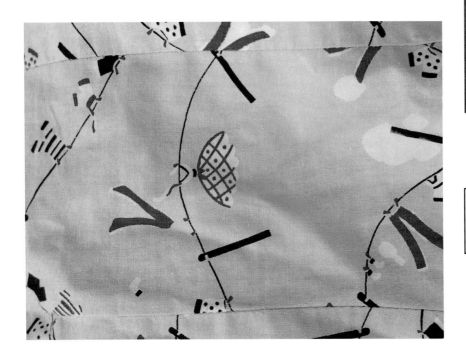

Early play clothes airing on the line in sunny California. The fabric detail shows great charm, as does model Elizabeth Haskett. Her romper is by Candy Jones, circa 1950.

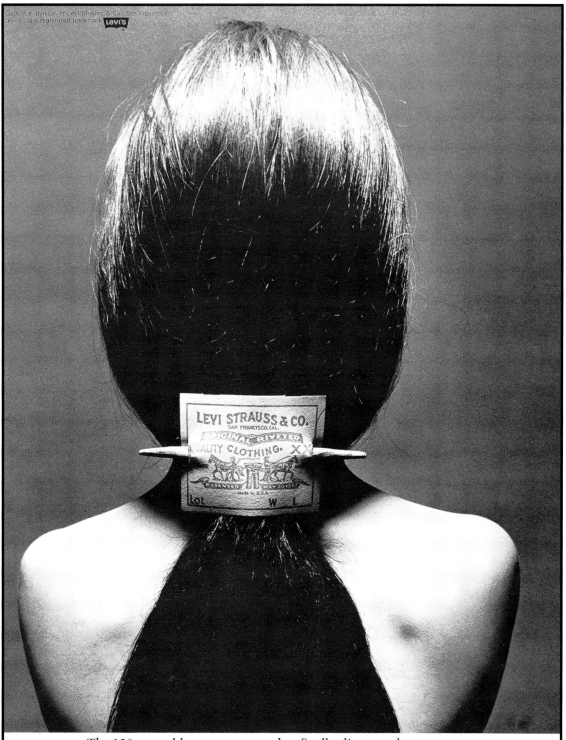

The 120 year old pants company has finally discovered women.

Levi's for Gals

The iconic power of Levi's leather patch was recognized in a 1970s ad campaign that launched *Levi's for Gals*: "The 120 year old pants company has finally discovered women."

On the whole, Americans were the first to produce sportswear. By the 1940s, the idea had coalesced into a functional design ethic that still seems modern today. But the industry was dug from the mines of California a century earlier, like nuggets of gold in the guise of blue denim. After all, when Levi Strauss hawked his overalls to the '49ers it marked the first time in history that a business had been founded on the manufacture of garments meant to be worn outdoors, for a specific and utilitarian purpose.

In this book, we will explore the industry as it developed in California from the 1930s through the 1970s, with emphasis on clothing and textile designs suffused with the sunshine spirit. There are few dresses and no ensembles, with the exception of hostess wear for pool and patio. We will look at the major swimwear companies Catalina, Cole, and Rose Marie Reid, as well as sportswear leaders like Koret and Alice of California.

Throughout, we will see how new developments in fabric technology have inspired designers, and have been stimulated by them in return. And we will pay tribute to that most western of fabrics, blue denim, which has made a lasting impression on casual clothing design, from ranch dressing to rock star dressing room.

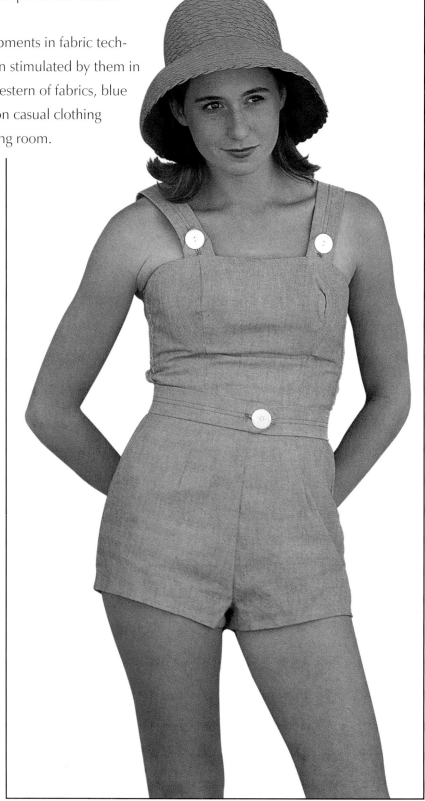

Kim Davidson romps in pink denim by John Weitz of California, circa 1965. *Courtesy, Cheap Thrills.*

Opposite page
Although the label is Campus Casual, by today's standard the look is *not*. Elizabeth Haskett looks dressed for a board meeting in this rayon blend coat suit, but it was marketed to ladies who lunched, circa 1955.

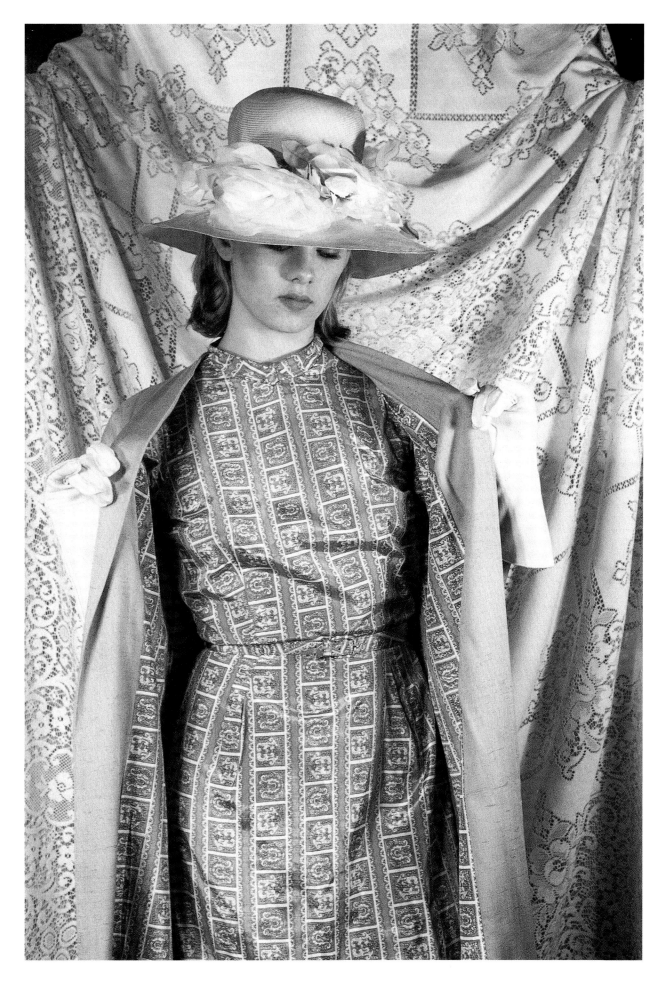

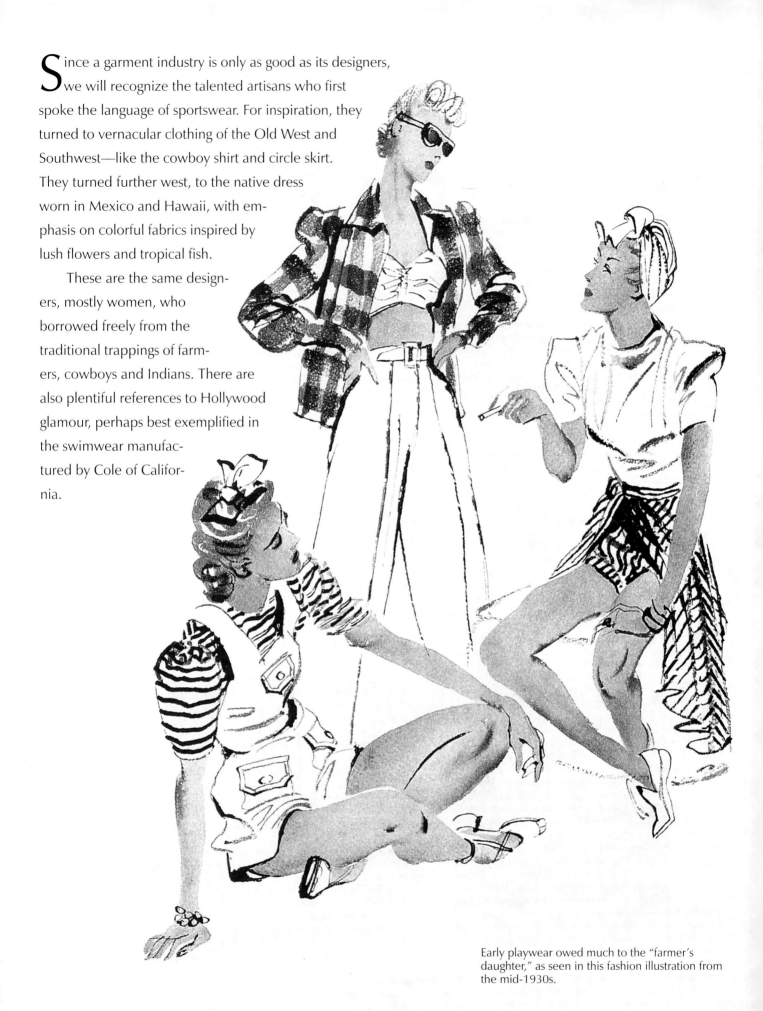

Since a garment industry is only as good as its designers, we will recognize the talented artisans who first spoke the language of sportswear. For inspiration, they turned to vernacular clothing of the Old West and Southwest—like the cowboy shirt and circle skirt. They turned further west, to the native dress worn in Mexico and Hawaii, with emphasis on colorful fabrics inspired by lush flowers and tropical fish.

These are the same designers, mostly women, who borrowed freely from the traditional trappings of farmers, cowboys and Indians. There are also plentiful references to Hollywood glamour, perhaps best exemplified in the swimwear manufactured by Cole of California.

Early playwear owed much to the "farmer's daughter," as seen in this fashion illustration from the mid-1930s.

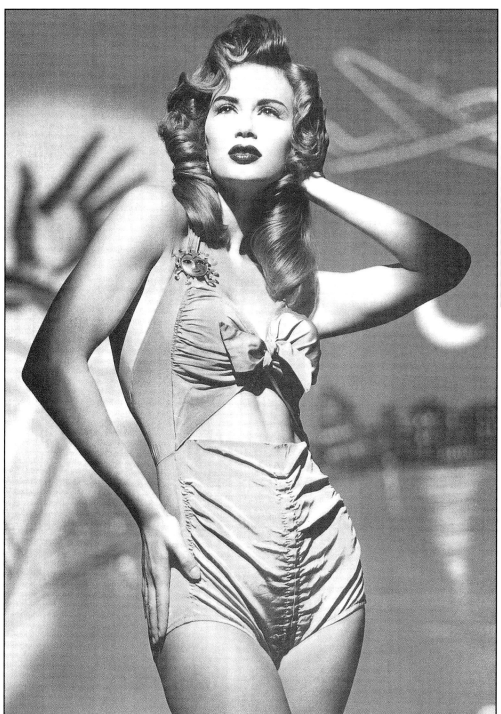

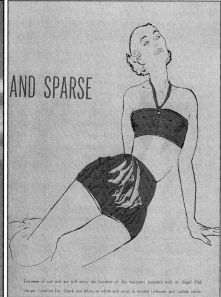

Angel Fish animate a surf 'n sun outfit offered by Catalina in 1948. The fabric is knit Jacquard with Lastex for stretch. It came in black and white, or white and coral.

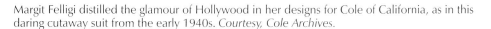

Margit Felligi distilled the glamour of Hollywood in her designs for Cole of California, as in this daring cutaway suit from the early 1940s. *Courtesy, Cole Archives.*

The result was a strong mixture of culture and attitude forged on the anvils of gold fever, iron plowshares, and silver screen. The design alloy that emerged must be recognized as pure California Casual.

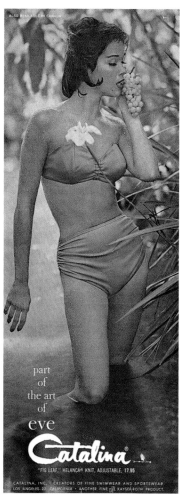

This 1940s two-piecer blends tropical jungle with paradise lost. According to Catalina it's "Part of the Art of Eve."

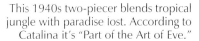

chapter 1
THE PIONEERS

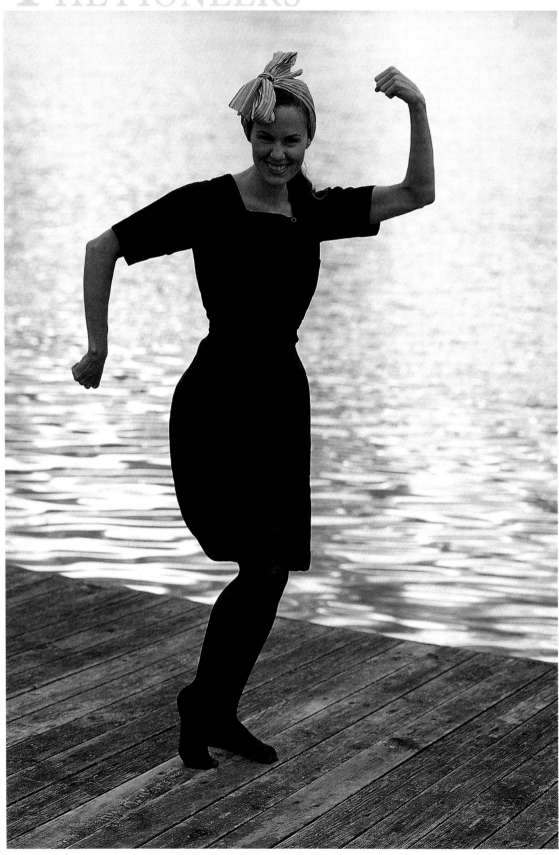

Naomi Duffy shows some muscle in a black cotton gym suit from the early 1900s (no label). *Courtesy, Doreen Sinclair.*

"By the 1940s, a California style had developed that was becoming popular throughout the country. People everywhere were looking at the fashions worn by the Hollywood stars, and the Hollywood stars were often buying their clothes from local designers whose work was suited to the West Coast life-style. The California fashion industry was setting trends in a new area of casual clothing, sportswear. Outdoor sports, which became popular during the late nineteenth century, required special clothing. This attire had to allow freedom of movement and was expected to be stylish as well."

—Edward Maeder, curator for the Los Angeles County Museum of Art, 1986.

Wealthy Americans, like their European counterparts, have long loved the sporting life (think of hunt balls, horse shows and yacht clubs), but leisure sports were not accessible to the middle class until relatively recently. This cultural shift had its origins in the Industrial Revolution, when technology, and the transition from farm to city life, made a six-day workweek feasible.

Moral pundits publicly debated over the potentially harmful effects of so much free time on the hands of blue collar workers. Ultimately, there was a broad-based revival of interest in the ancient Greek fitness triad of mind, body, and spirit—ushering gymnastics into the schools, and athletics onto the streets.

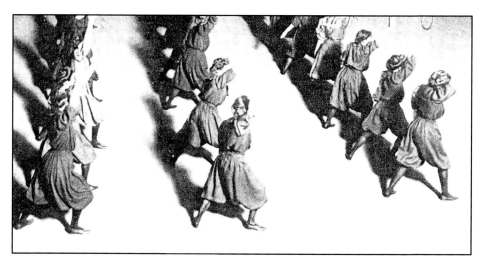

Baggy bloomers were typically worn with woolen hose and leather shoes, as shown in this photo of a 1900s gym class.

Good Sports

There were differences in the degree of sporting activities deemed suitable for men and women, stemming from Victorian views of womanly piety. The reproductive functions were seen as a divinely-ordered divide between the level of physical exertion that women and men could safely undertake.

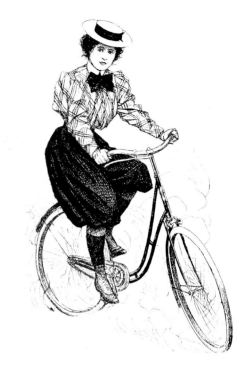

Women were ensconced in layers of clothing for every sport, ostensibly to protect their modesty and propriety. The practical effect was to hamper their very safety. Skirts could tangle in the wheels of a bicycle, or cause a hiker to slip on the rocks; corsets caused fainting spells on the croquet lawn, and heavy woolen suits could easily pull a bather under the surf.

The dress reform movement that began in the mid-1800s finally began to succeed when active women demanded freedom from restrictive overskirts, corsets, and bustles. The first real test of rational dress came with the immense popularity of cycling in the 1890s.

An early bicycling costume, circa 1890.

Once manufacturers learned how to mass produce chain-driven wheels of equal size, it seemed everyone must ride the new "safety bicycles" about town and country. This paved the way for other forms of public exercise, like golf and tennis. Soon, private clubs were installing greens, and municipalities were dedicating public beaches to meet the demand of sports enthusiasts from coast-to-coast.

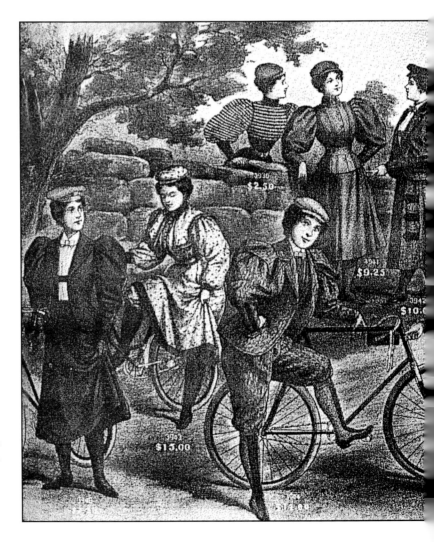

Adventurous women wore bloomers; their timid sisters wore shortened skirts.

14

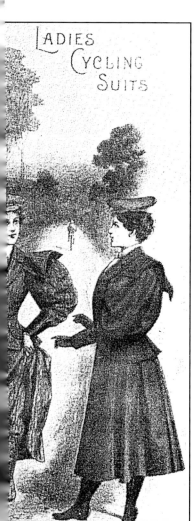

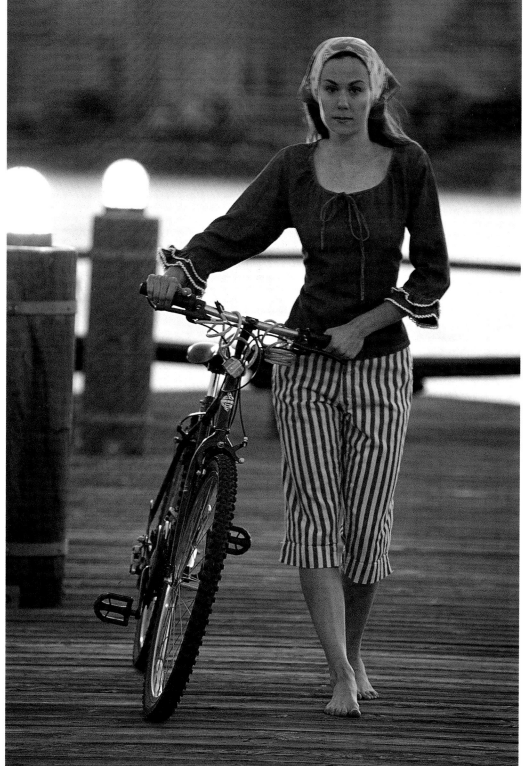

By the mid-century women were free to don shorts for biking, like these in red-and-white denim (no label, circa 1960). The blouse is not vintage—nor is the bike! *Author's collection.*

By the 1920s, a fitness craze was sweeping the country, leaving the nascent garment industry unsure of a response. At first, there was little distinction between types of sportswear. Even swimsuits were just a slightly briefer version of the blouse-and-bloomers ensemble with which schools outfitted their gym students. In 1876, a woman's swimsuit could weigh twenty pounds when wet, rendering actual *swimming* impossible.

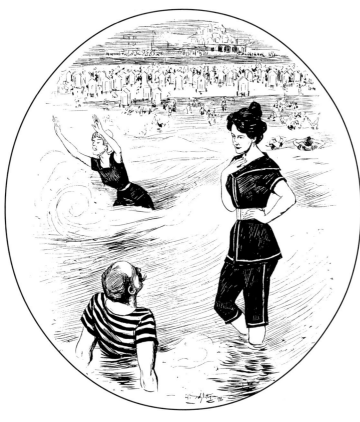

"By the sea, by the sea, by the beautiful sea."
Flirting in the surf is a hundred-year-old art.

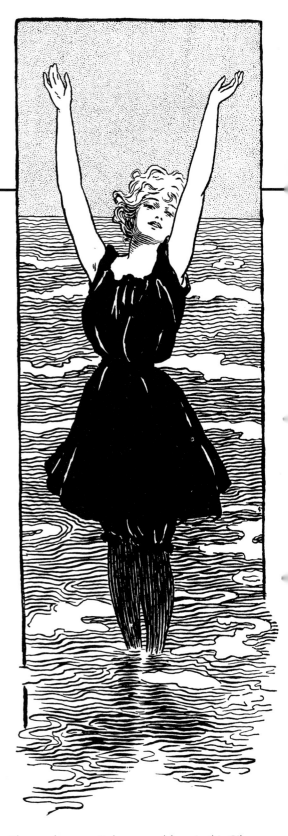

The wool serge suit shows good form in this Gibson Girl illustration.

Gantner of California had its origins in the San Francisco knitwear firm, Gantner-Mattern Co. It was founded by J.O. Gantner and G.A. Mattern, both executives with Pfister Knitting, which had been supplying swimwear to the nation since 1876. They bought out the knittery after it was damaged in the great San Francisco earthquake, forming their own company in 1906.

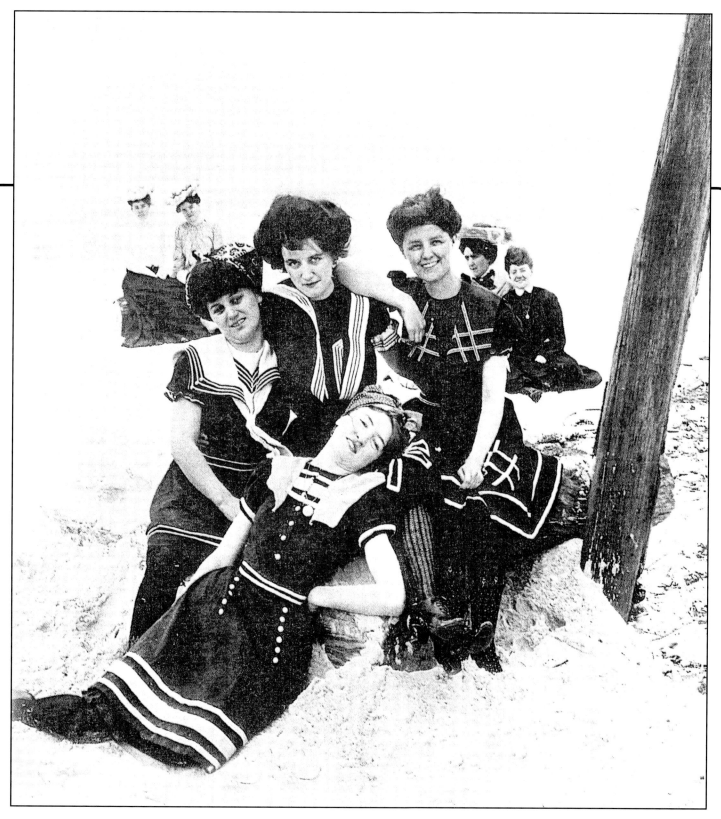

In 1906, these woolen bathing suits were daring; to the modern eye, they seem restrictive. *Courtesy, Library of Congress.*

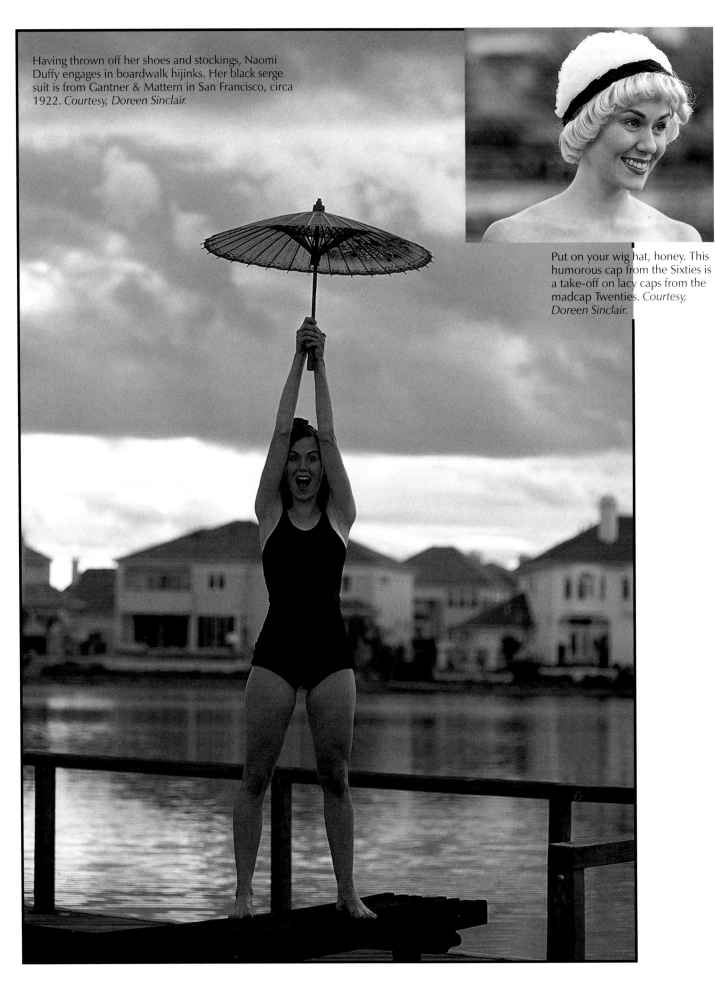

Having thrown off her shoes and stockings, Naomi Duffy engages in boardwalk hijinks. Her black serge suit is from Gantner & Mattern in San Francisco, circa 1922. *Courtesy, Doreen Sinclair.*

Put on your wig hat, honey. This humorous cap from the Sixties is a take-off on lacy caps from the madcap Twenties. *Courtesy, Doreen Sinclair.*

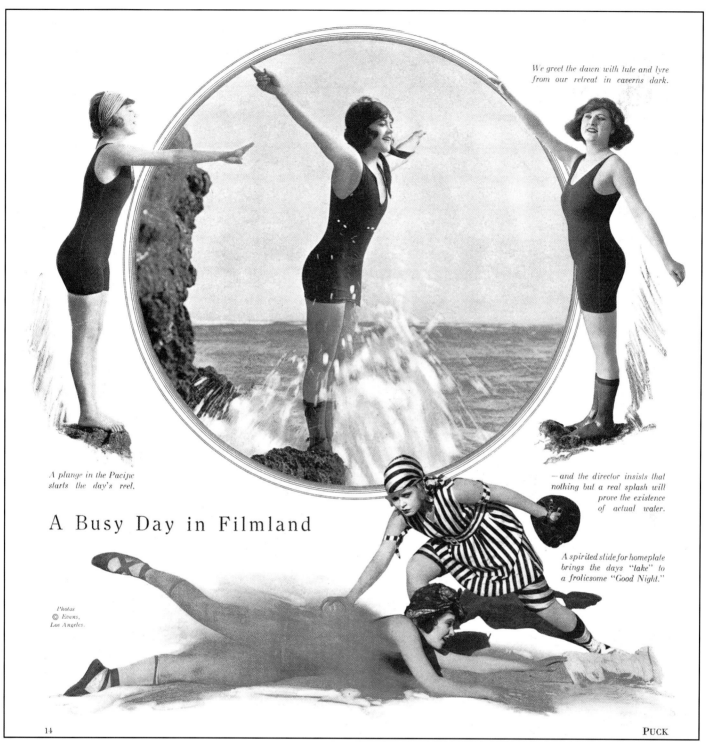

We greet the dawn with lute and lyre
from our retreat in caverns dark.

A plunge in the Pacific
starts the day's reel.

A Busy Day in Filmland

—and the director insists that
nothing but a real splash will
prove the existence
of actual water.

A spirited slide for homeplate
brings the days "take" to
a frolicsome "Good Night."

Photos
© Evans,
Los Angeles.

PUCK

This bathing beauty feature, from the June 1918 issue of *Puck* magazine, was themed around "A Busy Day in Filmland." Note the swimsuit-clad baseball players on the bottom. *Photos by Evans of Los Angeles.*

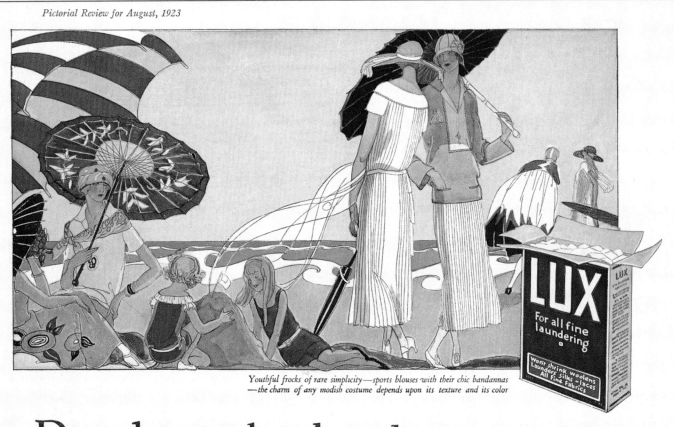

*Youthful frocks of rare simplicity—sports blouses with their chic bandannas
—the charm of any modish costume depends upon its texture and its color*

Don't let careless laundering
shrink or fade them ~ *Washed this way*
your sport clothes keep their texture and their color

Before there was a sportswear industry, both men and women cobbled together the least restrictive items in their wardrobes. Many early sports costumes borrowed from the ease of resortwear. A man might wear his white woolen slacks for golf; his wife might choose her white eyelet dress, with a shortened skirt, for lawn tennis.

Lux promoted its gentle soap for laundering "sports clothes" in the August 1923 issue of *Pictorial Review*. This beach scene portrays ladies in "youthful frocks of rare simplicity—sports blouses with chic bandannas."

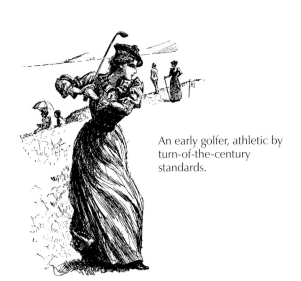

An early golfer, athletic by turn-of-the-century standards.

Opposite page
A golf dress advertised by Royal of California in November 1949.

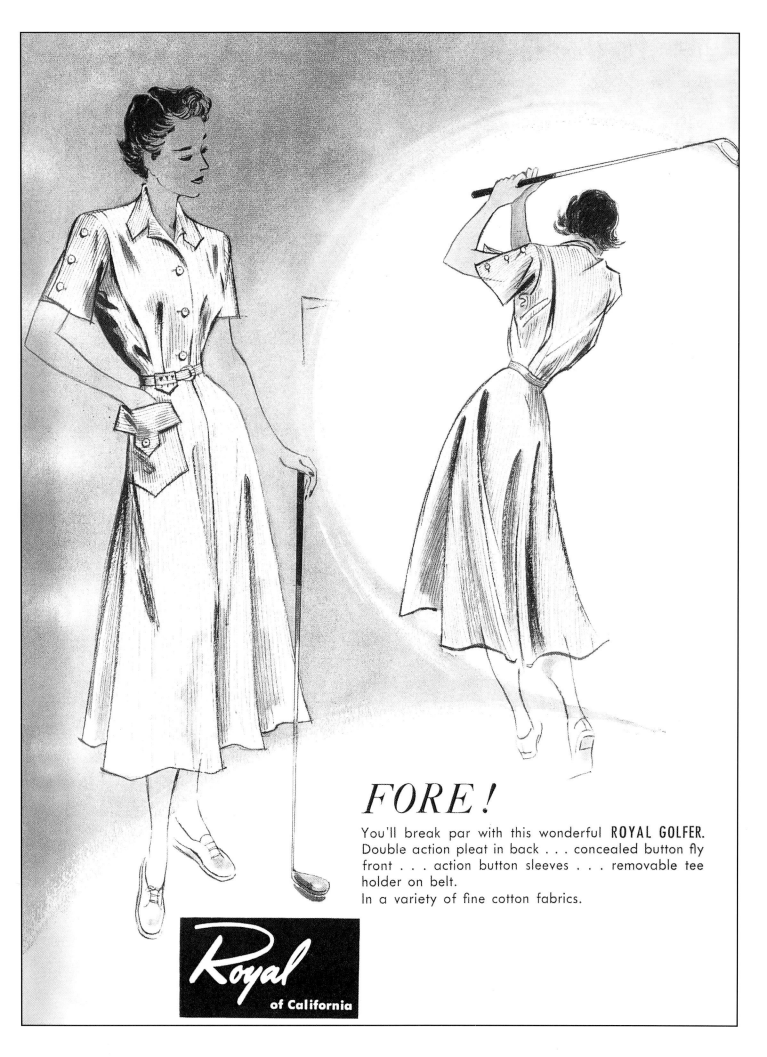

FORE!

You'll break par with this wonderful ROYAL GOLFER. Double action pleat in back . . . concealed button fly front . . . action button sleeves . . . removable tee holder on belt.
In a variety of fine cotton fabrics.

Royal
of California

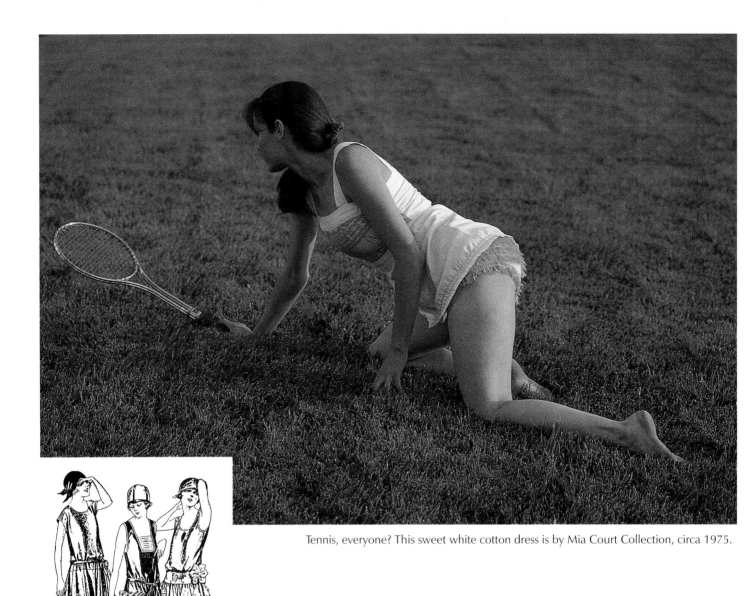

Tennis, everyone? This sweet white cotton dress is by Mia Court Collection, circa 1975.

Four bathing suits and a tennis dress with sass and style, for Spring 1922.

The invention of man-made fiber was instrumental in the development of sportswear. As when Levi Strauss ingeniously used tent fabric to outfit gold miners, manufacturers began to convert existing mills and workrooms to produce clothing that was flexible and reliable enough to meet the demands of sports enthusiasts.

By the 1920s, elastic yarns were used for swimwear; by the 1940s, stretch panels were set into jersey golf dresses, for ease. As the genre developed, bold fasteners were selected for speed, and bright patterns were used just for fun.

Pockets were a great convenience for active women, and were often integrated into early casual designs. According to Richard Martin, writing for the Metropolitan Museum of Art's *American Ingenuity* catalog: "Absence of pockets is a real social handicap long perpetuated in women's fashion . . . [leaving them] unable to participate in the commerce and conveniences of modern life." Given their utility, it's no wonder that women designers routinely stitched pockets into sports clothes, along with special tabs and belts for carrying gear.

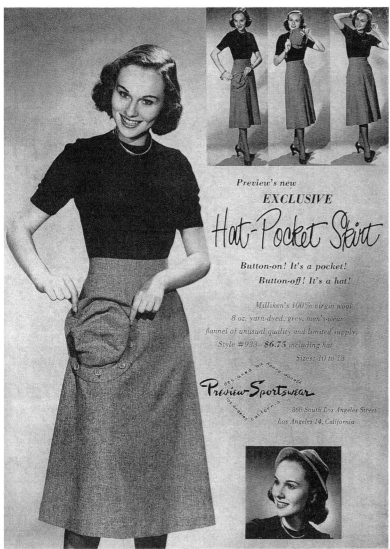

Preview's new
EXCLUSIVE
Hot-Pocket Skirt

Button-on! It's a pocket!
Button-off! It's a hat!

Milliken's 100% virgin wool,
8 oz. yarn-dyed, grey, men's-wear
flannel of unusual quality and limited supply.
Style #933—$6.75 including hat
Sizes: 10 to 18

Preview Sportswear

860 South Los Angeles Street
Los Angeles 14, California

Hot-Pocket Skirt as advertised by Preview Sportswear of California, January 1951. Women could stow their stuff, or shade their heads. "Button-on! It's a pocket! Button-off! It's a hat!"

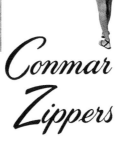

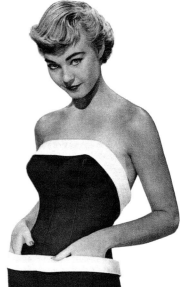

Conmar
Zippers

GUARANTEED FLAWLESS

When your social security depends on
a zipper's lock action . . . be grateful for
the stay-put Conmar. Conmar defies
gravity . . . it won't slide, come high dive
or seaside calisthenics . . .
lies flat as a seam, whatever your pleasure.
No wonder you'll find Conmar zippers
on America's finest swimsuits.

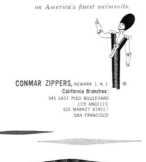

CONMAR ZIPPERS, NEWARK 1, N. J.
California Branches:
945 EAST PICO BOULEVARD
LOS ANGELES
420 MARKET STREET
SAN FRANCISCO

Pragmatic and prolific, Rose Marie Reid built pockets into many swimsuit designs, as seen in this 1951 promotion by Conmar Zippers.

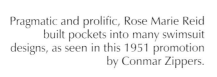

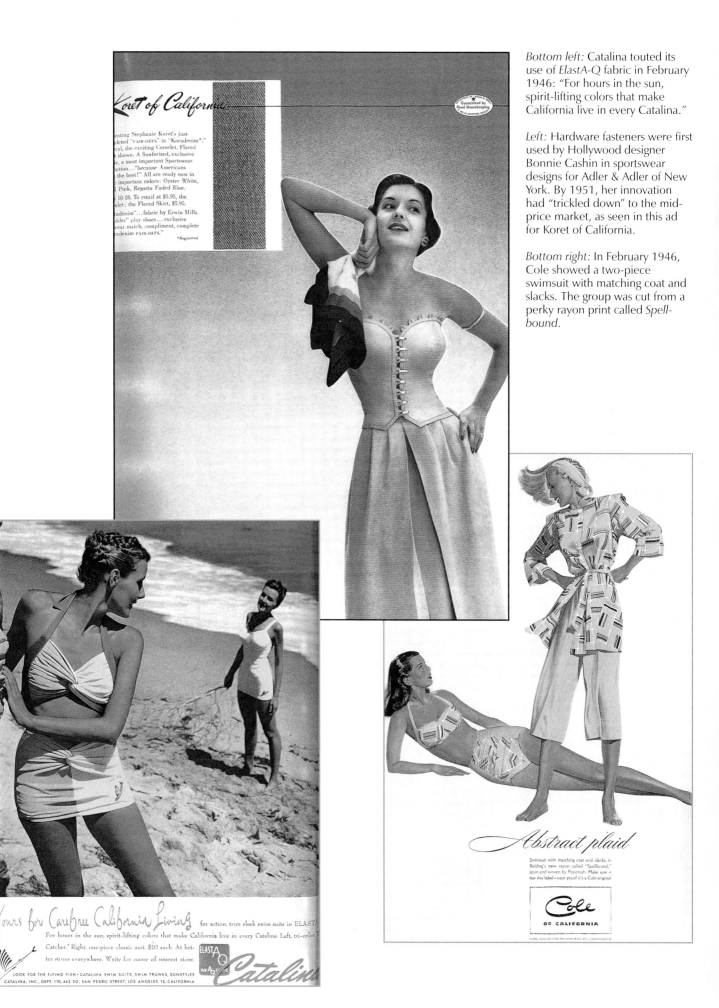

Bottom left: Catalina touted its use of *ElastA-Q* fabric in February 1946: "For hours in the sun, spirit-lifting colors that make California live in every Catalina."

Left: Hardware fasteners were first used by Hollywood designer Bonnie Cashin in sportswear designs for Adler & Adler of New York. By 1951, her innovation had "trickled down" to the mid-price market, as seen in this ad for Koret of California.

Bottom right: In February 1946, Cole showed a two-piece swimsuit with matching coat and slacks. The group was cut from a perky rayon print called *Spellbound*.

Koret of California

enting Stephanie Koret's just-
pleted "PAIR-OFFS" in "Koradenim*,"
cal, the exciting Corselet, Flared
k shown. A Sanforized, exclusive
e, a most important Sportswear
ption..."because Americans
the best!" All are ready now in
important colors: Oyster White,
l Pink, Regatta Faded Blue.
10-18. To retail at $5.95, the
elet; the Flared Skirt, $5.95.
adenim"...fabric by Erwin Mills.
bbler" play shoes...exclusive
wear match, compliment, complete
radenim PAIR-OFFS."

*Registered

Yours for Carefree California Living for action, trim sleek swim suits in ELASTA
For hours in the sun, spirit-lifting colors that make California live in every Catalina. Left, tri-color
Catcher." Right, one-piece classic suit. $10 each. At bet-
ter stores everywhere. Write for name of nearest store.

LOOK FOR THE FLYING FISH • CATALINA SWIM SUITS, SWIM TRUNKS, SUNSTYLES
CATALINA, INC., DEPT. 110, 443 SO. SAN PEDRO STREET, LOS ANGELES 13, CALIFORNIA

ELASTA Q
AN Q FABRIC

Catalina

Abstract plaid

Swimsuit with matching coat and slacks, in
Belding's new rayon called "Spellbound,"
spun and woven by Ponemah. Make sure it
has this label—your proof it's a Cole original

Cole
OF CALIFORNIA

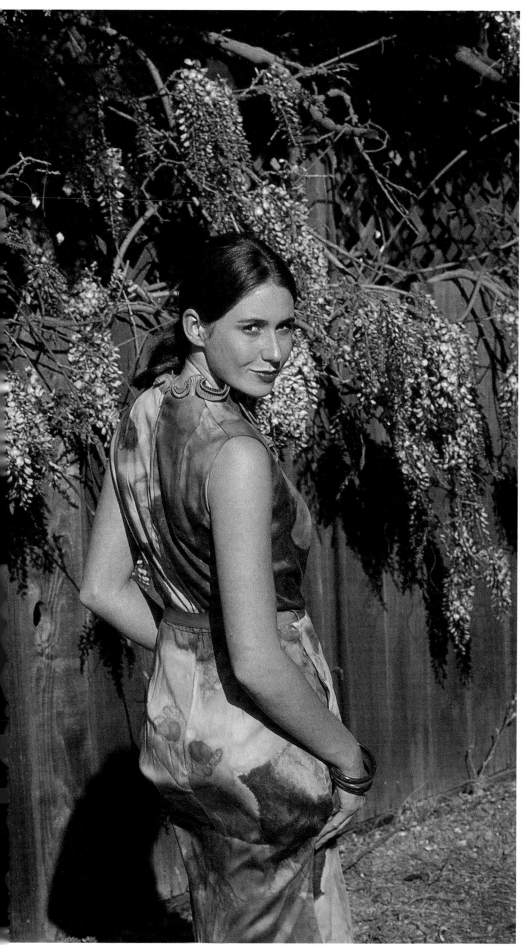

These days, the image of a well-toned woman is readily accepted as feminine and alluring. Such was not the case mid-century, when even active woman were expected to be curvaceous. As a result, early swimsuits were often styled like ballgowns, and vintage sportswear designed for day now seems suitable for evening.

In the 1950s-1970s, Alice featured a *Polynesian* division with loungewear cut from vivid tropical prints. The gown shown on Kim Davidson is fine for summer evenings, now.

The Artisans

Unique in the rag trade, female designers soon outdistanced their male counterparts in the race for quality sportswear. In New York, it was Claire McCardell and Clare Potter, Carolyn Schnurer and Vera Maxwell. In California, it was artisans like Louella Ballerino, who infused her clothing designs with a folklore reference; and Juli Lynne Charlot, who created the felt circle skirt. The distaff baton *did* pass to one man, and a Californian at that: internationally-acclaimed designer Rudi Gernreich.

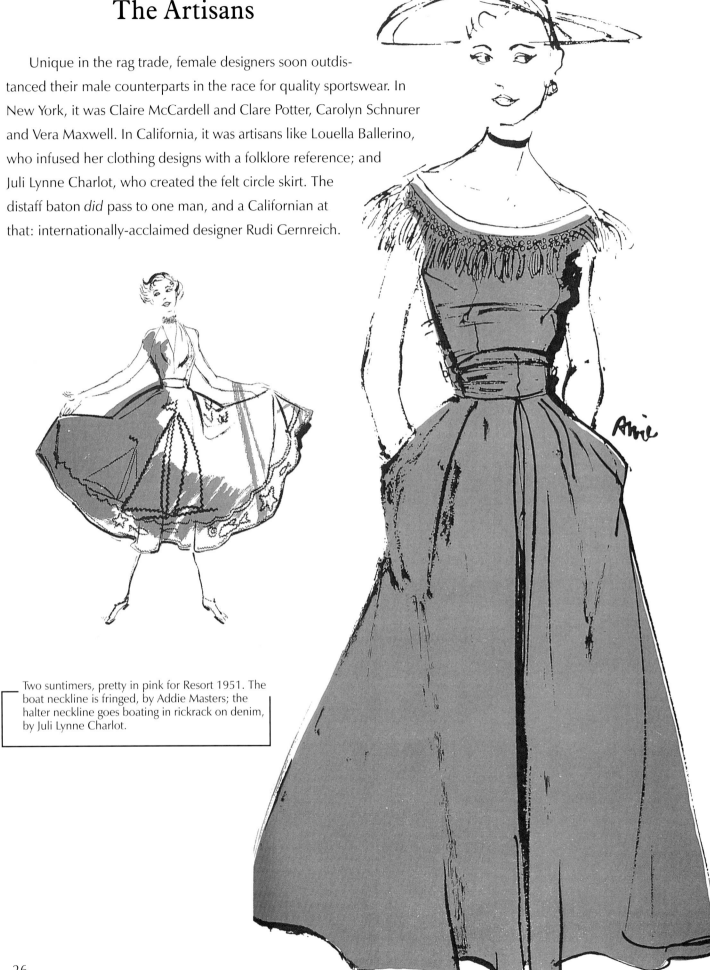

Two suntimers, pretty in pink for Resort 1951. The boat neckline is fringed, by Addie Masters; the halter neckline goes boating in rickrack on denim, by Juli Lynne Charlot.

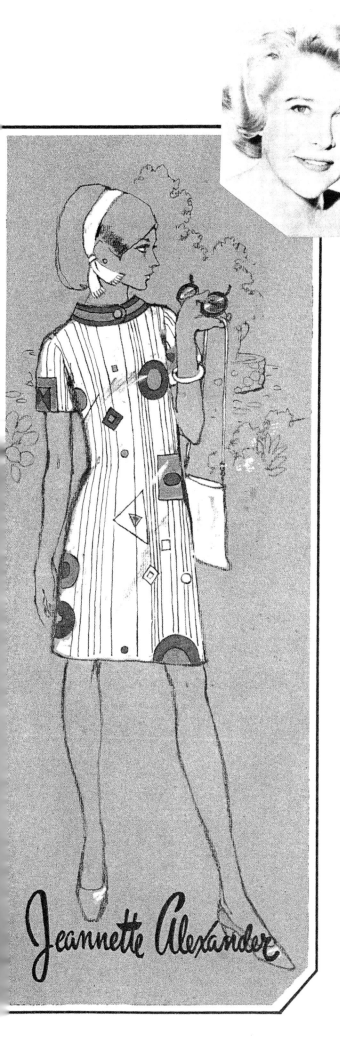

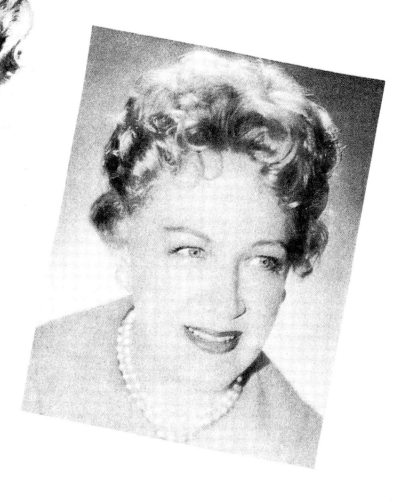

Jeanette Alexander & Peggy Hunt

Peggy Hunt began her career designing party clothes for her little girl Jeanette. From there, she grew into junior fashions and matured into a womanly line of after-five dresses and evening gowns. It was only natural that a grown-up Jeanette Alexander would follow in her creative mother's footsteps. At first, she designed for the Peggy Hunt label. Then, in the 1960s, she created her own company with a quality junior line. Her designs were marked by zippy cotton prints for day, and hip metallics for night, usually cut in a simple princess or sheath silhouette.

By the 1960s, Hunt and Alexander liked to partner their advertising, as shown in this example from the *California Stylist* of August 1968.

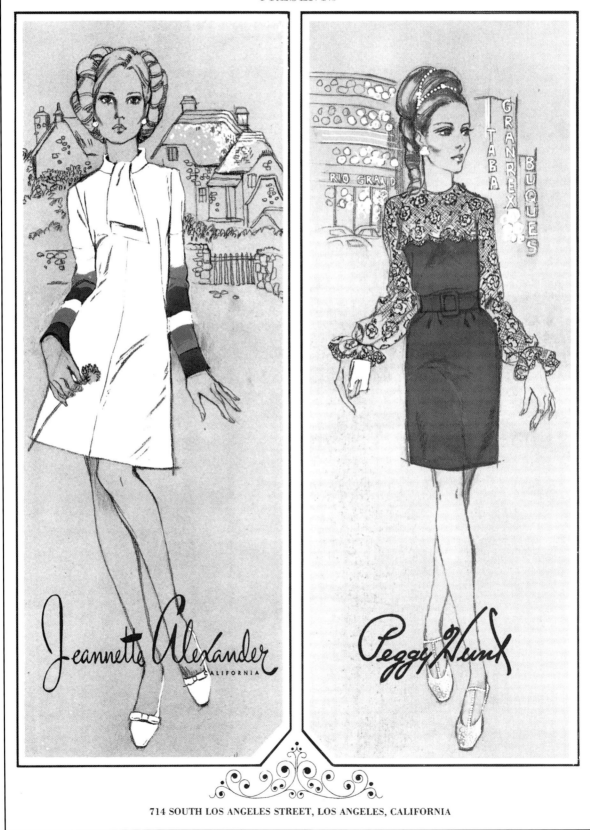

JEANNETTE HYLAND INC.
PRESENTS

Jeannette Alexander
CALIFORNIA

Peggy Hunt

714 SOUTH LOS ANGELES STREET, LOS ANGELES, CALIFORNIA

Louella Ballerino

Like a fashion archeologist, Louella Ballerino incorporated traditional regional styles into a unique and functional line of casual clothing. As an

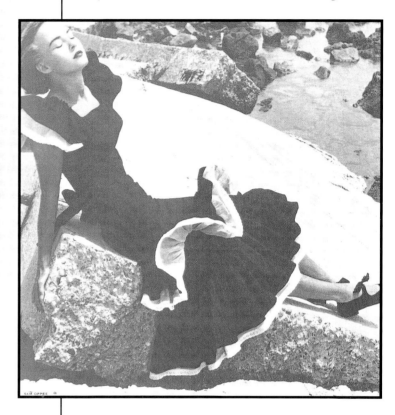

Above left: The practical pocket turns into an element of design on this skirt, as featured in the *California Stylist* in August 1950: "Louella Ballerino outlines a giant diamond of a pocket with black braid, traces a series of concentric lines with rows of glittering jet."

Above right: A flouncy two-piece sundress in black cotton poplin, popped over a white lawn petticoat. This Western charmer was designed by Ballerino in the mid-1940s.

art major at the University of Southern California, she studied under Andre-Ani, a designer at Metro-Goldwyn-Mayer in Hollywood. Ballerino began her career by working in a custom dress shop and selling sketches to various garment manufacturers.

Ballerino also taught fashion theory at the Frank Wiggins Trade School in Los Angeles. In one interview, she divulged a unique teaching philosophy: "I always told my students that they couldn't expect to be really original. After all, there are just so many colors in the world, and so many lines; and everything they could conceive of had, somewhere, sometime, been done before."

Rather a bleak outlook, until Ballerino explained how she told students to "create new styles by applying their minds to the adaptation of already-existing things." As with the very modern notion of reviving vintage styles until they are suitable for life in the year 2000, so it was in 1930. What's old is new again.

This was the same approach Ballerino applied when she opened her own design firm. By the late 1930s, she was interpreting European peasant dress in the form of Dutch-boy trousers, and South American folk costume cut into embroidered blouses. In the latter collection, Ballerino used fabric bands handwoven in Peru as an important design detail. She's credited with adapting the peasant apron and dirndl skirt for streetwear, decades before the craze for peasant dressing stormed America in the 1960s. She was also one of the first to design mother-daughter outfits in the postwar years, establishing a fashion parable of strong family values.

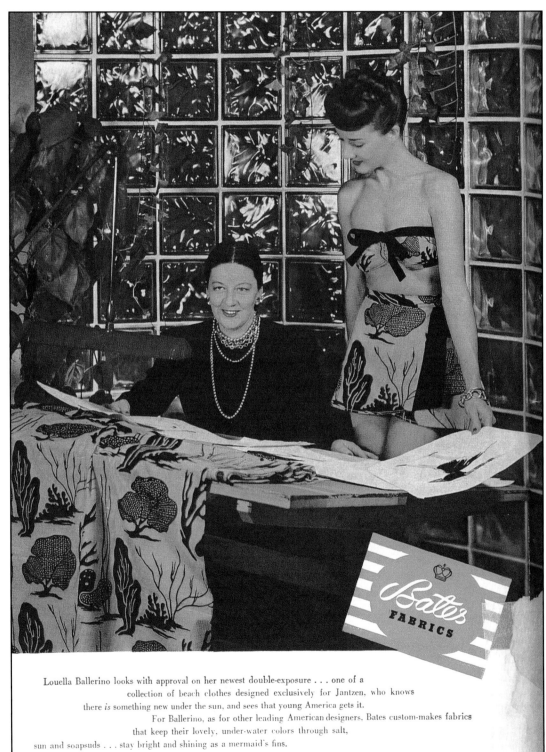

Ballerino is shown approving a sea-fern pattern by Bates Fabrics in this advertisement from the February 1, 1946 issue of *Vogue*.

Louella Ballerino looks with approval on her newest double-exposure . . . one of a collection of beach clothes designed exclusively for Jantzen, who knows there *is* something new under the sun, and sees that young America gets it. For Ballerino, as for other leading American designers, Bates custom-makes fabrics that keep their lovely, under-water colors through salt, sun and soapsuds . . . stay bright and shining as a mermaid's fins.

In the mid-1940s, Ballerino designed beach clothes for Jantzen, a Seattle-based swim and sportswear company. A major element of this outstanding collection lay in the custom prints she ordered from Bates Fabrics with inspiration from Hawaii, Africa, and Polynesia (even, apparently, from Victorian America).

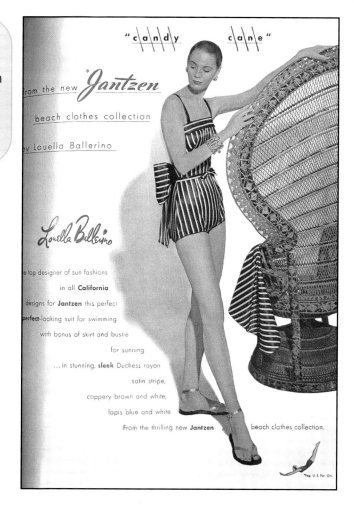

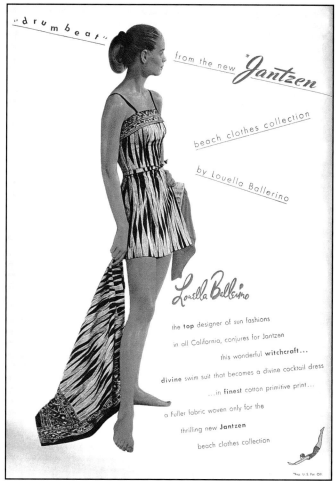

Above & above right: The *Drumbeat* and *Candy Cane* designs, as advertised for Resort 1947.

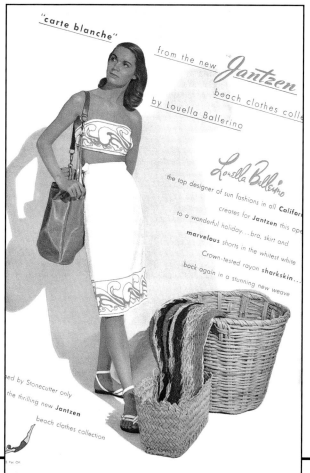

In the *Carte Blanche* design, Ballerino paired a bra top with a wraparound skirt or shorts (not shown). The white fabric, a special-order rayon sharkskin, has a delightful sea-green wave border.

Agnes Barrett

Agnes Barrett is one of the original members of the "eight designing women" who formed the merchandising group Affiliated
Fashionists. This group had quite a concentration of casual clothing
designers—the roster included Louella Ballerino, De De Johnson and
Addie Masters, along with Barrett.

Barrett is credited with producing the first *broomstick* skirt in
1940. It's a pretty and practical style, which has been revived just
about every decade since then. It took months to execute this entirely
original design, which finally emerged only after Barrett tied a wet
skirt around a broomstick to form a cascade of wrinkles flowing
evenly from waist to hem. The skirt can be washed and wrung dry,
and, like its haute couture silk cousins from the house of Mario
Fortuny, it can be packed like a knotted strand of rope.

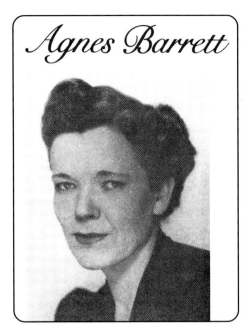

Agnes Barrett.

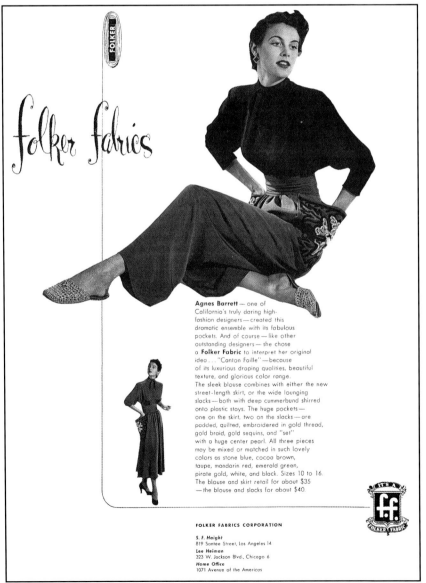

Luxurious separates by Barrett.

This Agnes Barrett original was promoted by Folker Fabrics Corp. in the
California Stylist of November 1949. The
ad detailed each outfit:

"The sleek blouse combines with
either the new street-length skirt, or the
wide lounging slacks—both with deep
cummerbund shirred onto plastic stays.
The huge pockets—one on the skirt, two
on the slacks—are padded, quilted,
embroidered in gold thread, gold braid,
gold sequins, and 'set' with a huge center
pearl. All three pieces may be mixed or
matched in such lovely colors as stone
blue, cocoa brown, taupe, mandarin red,
emerald green, pirate gold, white and
black. Sizes 10 to 16. The blouse and skirt
retail for about $35—the blouse and
slacks for about $40."

As seen by this description, buyers could
choose from a wide range of practical colors
and real-women sizes (the vintage size range
10-16 is equivalent to our 8-12). The
"mixed and matched" concept was one of
many new ideas pioneered by American
sportswear designers.

Bonnie Cashin

California born-and-bred, Bonnie Cashin moved to New York City in the early 1930s to study ballet. Before long, she was enrolled in the Art Student's League and working as a costume designer for the Roxy Theater. In 1937, she began free-lancing for the Seventh Avenue sportswear giant Adler & Adler, where she championed separates dressing.

In 1943, Cashin was lured to Hollywood with a job offer from the costume department at 20th Century Fox. Cashin worked as a movie designer for the next six years, dressing Gene Tierney in *Laura* (1944) and the principals in *Anna and the King of Siam* (1946).

She returned to New York in 1949 in order to found her own garment business, The Knittery. The very next year, she was awarded the Coty American Fashion Critic's Award on behalf of "her gay and witty approach to sport and street clothes [that] brought new vitality to fashion."

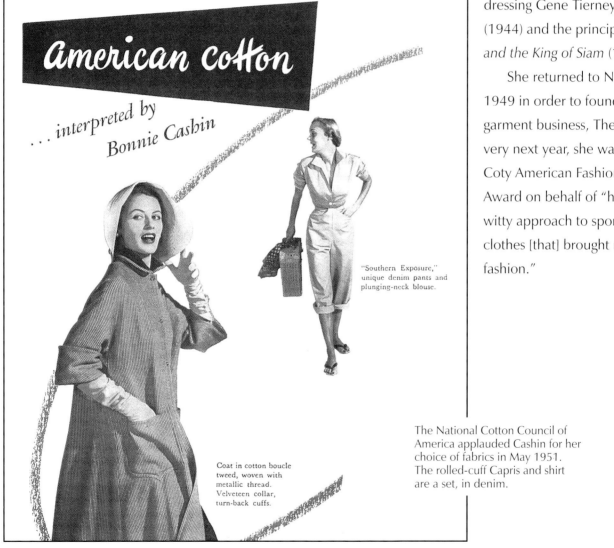

american cotton

...interpreted by Bonnie Cashin

"Southern Exposure," unique denim pants and plunging-neck blouse.

Coat in cotton boucle tweed, woven with metallic thread. Velveteen collar, turn-back cuffs.

The National Cotton Council of America applauded Cashin for her choice of fabrics in May 1951. The rolled-cuff Capris and shirt are a set, in denim.

Cashin is credited with many innovations, including the bandanna apron in 1956 and paper dresses in 1966. She mixed fabrics fearlessly—pairing leather with wool, suede with doubleknit, and tweed with mohair. Perhaps her most resourceful design contribution was with *fasteners*. She substituted luggage toggles in place of buttons on a suit, and even used a dog leash hook to drape a layered skirt. With this background, it's only natural that she designed an outstanding line of functional handbags for Coach, in the 1960s.

Hearkening back to her West Coast roots, Cashin infused many designs with a Pacific Rim sensibility, as in her Kimono-shaped jackets for Fall 1964. And she referenced the Southwest in signature woolen ponchos, season after season.

Juli Lynne Charlot

The story of Juli Lynne Charlot is straight out of a Hollywood movie. Indeed, her first career was in show business—as a girl singer for Xavier Cugat, and as a "straight man" for the Marx Brothers.

Born Shirley Ann Agin, she learned fashion theory at the side of her mother, Betty Agin. At age five, she played with spools of thread in her mother's embroidery plant in Los Angeles. A few years later, the plant was producing a line of children's clothes inspired by little Shirley Ann.

Growing up, she studied art and design at Hollywood High School, and began modeling at age thirteen. There was a brief flurry of voice training toward a possible career in opera, which was soon abandoned in favor of dancing at the club Bal Tabarin in San Francisco. Shirley Ann was a nightclub performer at the tender age of sixteen! After adding singing to her repertoire, she was booked regularly at the swank Mark Hopkins hotel under the stage name "Juli Lynne." The local reviews were great—with the San Francisco newspapers taking as much notice of her costumes, which she designed herself, as her singing.

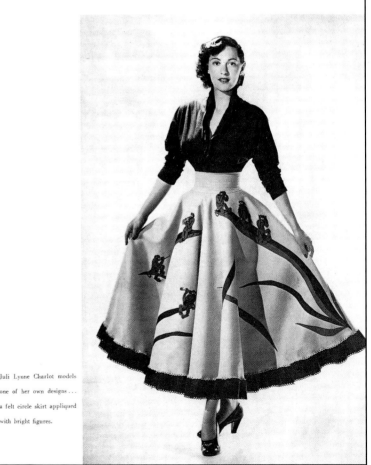

JULI LYNNE CHARLOT PERSONIFIES CALIFORNIA SPIRIT

Juli Lynne Charlot models one of her own designs . . . a felt circle skirt appliqued with bright figures.

Juli Lynn Charlot modeled her own designs, as seen in this ad from August 1950. It's her signature look of colorful appliqués on a felt circle skirt.

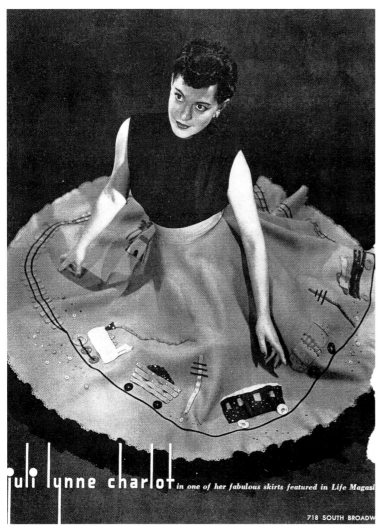

Juli Lynne Charlot *in one of her fabulous skirts featured in Life Magazi*

718 SOUTH BROADW

The "little engine that could" rounds the bend on a felt circle skirt. It's a good example of extravagant fashion by Charlot.

At about this same time, she was cast in two movies and worked between takes as a runway model. When the war began she performed for the troops, speaking for Harpo Marx and laughing at his brothers' gags onstage in a series of gigs arranged by the Hollywood Victory Committee. In 1946, she married Philip Charlot, a playwright and the son of a famous London producer.

Ironically, even though Charlot adopted her stage name from the female lead in *Showboat* (a role she had long coveted), she turned down the chance to play "Juli" because it would have meant a separation from her new husband. Young, beautiful, talented, romantic *and* newlywed: what more could a girl want? In this case, to express her talent without upsetting the domestic routine.

And so Charlot conceived the idea of designing a few festive skirts, perhaps selling them in a local store in time for the holiday season of 1947. Drawing on her schooling in embroidery, she created a felt circle skirt bordered with appliqués of Christmas trees. These skirts were an instant success, selling out the minute they went on display in the department store window.

Anecdotally, store buyers begged for more skirts to sell in the spring. When Charlot responded that she had no idea what design to use, since Christmas trees were no longer appropriate, they suggested: "Try anything! Try dogs!" From which inspiration the first poodle skirt was born, a design that is now recognized as an icon of Fifties fashion.

By the summer of 1950, Charlot was marketing her colorful skirts in about one hundred stores nationwide. She was promoted in a newspaper ad campaign by the retail giant Gimbel's, touting her in-store appearances as follows:

"Straight from the land where never is heard an unextravagant word . . . where oranges grow big as grapefruit and the sun shines 24 hours a day . . . where the newest fashion center in the world is a-borning . . . come Gimbel's California clothes [by] Juli Lynne Charlot. How original can clothes get!"

For all their extravagance of design, Charlot's skirts were meticulously tailored from quality fabrics. After her success with felt-on-felt appliqués—which were often three-dimensional—she ventured into special occasion skirts of taffeta and velvet, always with stitching or embroidery as a design detail. Charlot is also recognized as one of the first designers to pair skirts and sweaters as a daytime alternative to suits. A typical ensemble would consist of a pleated plaid skirt, coordinated with a sweater by embroidery and appliqués.

Rudi Gernreich

Rudi Gernreich arrived in Los Angeles in 1938 at age fourteen, a refugee from Nazi Germany, with no formal training in design and little command of the English language. But he had great artistic talent, and kept himself busy on the steamer from Europe by filling a notebook with design sketches. After taking a few art courses at Los Angeles City College he became a dancer for the Lester Horton Dance Troupe, then began designing their costumes.

Gernreich transitioned into textile design when he was hired by Hoffman Fabrics of California in 1945. His skill as a fashion designer became obvious when the bolts of cloth that he draped on mannequins for an ad campaign caused readers to ask where they could buy his clothes. That was in 1950, and Gernreich lost no time in designing a sample collection. Although he lacked the financial backing to begin mass production, he brought his samples to New York and caught the eye of *Harper's Bazaar* editor Diana Vreeland.

Back in Los Angeles and determined to start his own company, Gernreich approached top sportswear model Jimmy Mitchell in a store. He announced: "One day, you will be my fitting model." And she was, a few years later in 1951, when she helped get his line distributed through the trendy Beverly Hills boutique JAX. This led to a seven-year contract with the manufacturer Walter Bass, affiliated with Westwood Knitting Mills.

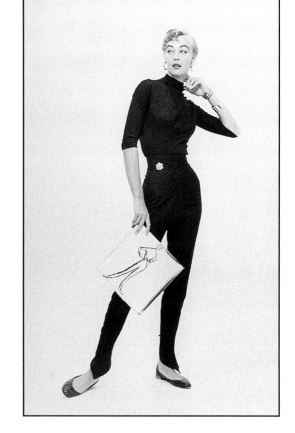

Jimmy Mitchell models an early pants set by Gernreich. Note his sketch, in her hand. *Courtesy, Jimmy Mitchell.*

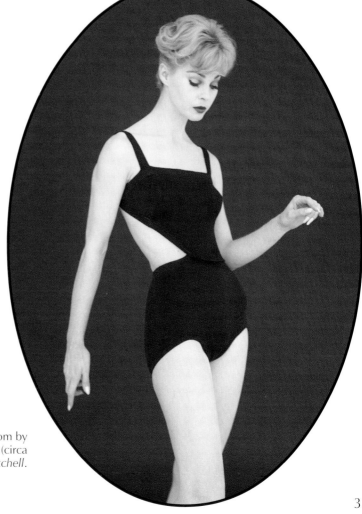

ernreich's collections were like nothing seen before when he exploded on the fashion scene in the 1950s. For a designer who couldn't use a needle and thread to sew on a button, he showed an amazing grasp of the properties of fabric—cutting felt so that it flared like a tunic *cum* tent, or using a lining like HyMo to trim the blouse of a pant set. In 1960, having just won the Coty American Fashion Critic's Award for sportswear, Gernreich started his own company.

His designs often reflected a spare, Oriental aesthetic. One of his most popular was a simple brocade jacket that he'd originally designed as a coat for the waiters at his favorite Chinese restaurant! Perhaps his most famous Oriental design was the "Obi" dress, cut from bold knits in mixed patterns. The knits were designed by Gernreich, and custom-ordered from his friend Harmon Juster who had left Westwood Knitting Mills to form Harmon Knits.

The unstructured cut of this black bombshell suit was a radical departure from the boned and wired styles prevalent in the early 1960s. *Courtesy, Jimmy Mitchell.*

Oh, baby! A bib top and diaper bottom by Rudi Gernreich for Harmon Knits (circa 1960). *Courtesy, Jimmy Mitchell.*

In the 1960s, Gernreich launched a series of themed looks inspired by the art of Beardsley one season, the artifacts of India the next. Among his many innovations, he introduced the top to toe look, including knit leggings coordinated with a mini-dress or tunic. Plus, he was a fabric mix-master, the first designer to put vinyl inserts into wool dresses for a startling peek-a-boo effect.

In 1963, Gernreich received the Coty American Fashion Critic's Award for high fashion. In 1967, he entered the Coty Hall of Fame next to such American design luminaries as Adrian, Claire McCardell, and Norman Norell.

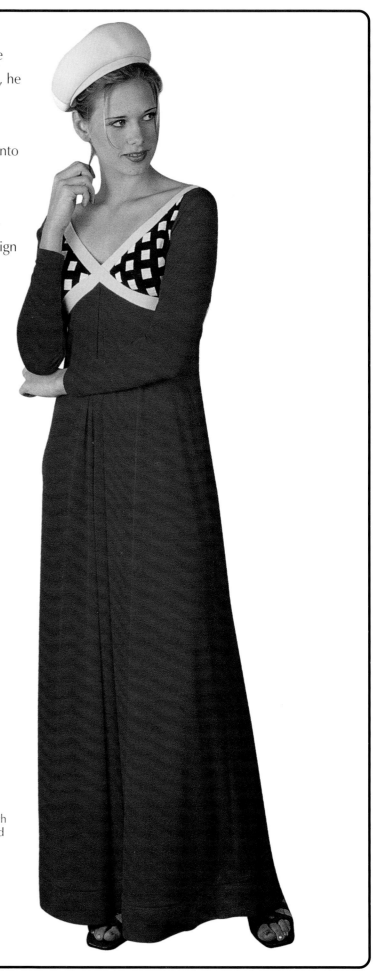

Gernreich's geometrics from the 1960s, modeled by Elizabeth Haskett. The label is Rudi Gernreich for Harmon Knits, the look is mixed knits.

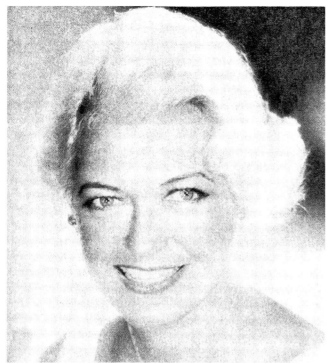

De De Johnson

In the 1930s, a young De De Johnson designed dance clothes with such flair that she was soon retained by a major Los Angeles dress firm. She eventually formed her own company, marketing to "the sophisticated woman's need for casual clothes." Her designs were marked by meticulous tailoring and an acute sense of proportion, giving them the ease and grace of a dance costume.

According to a *California Stylist* trade journal tribute in 1967: "De De Johnson is a classic name in California. It is synonymous with the casual life we lead in the west, with the kind of clothes that express our deepest con-

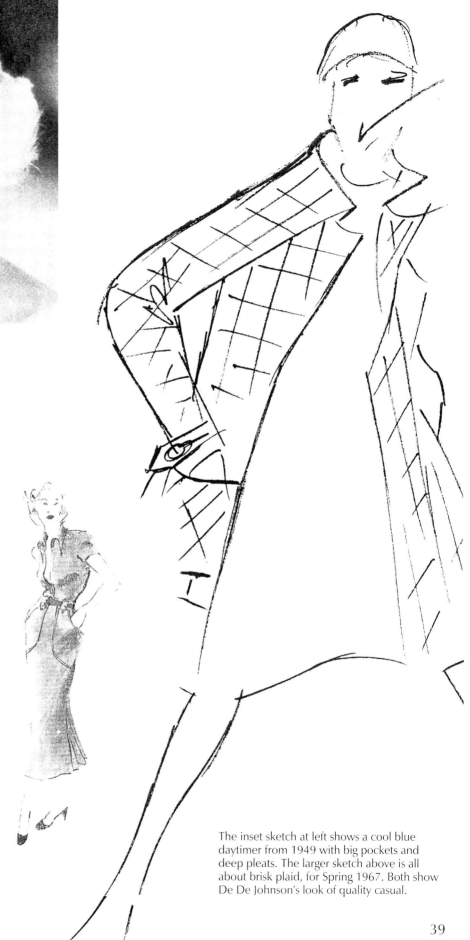

The inset sketch at left shows a cool blue daytimer from 1949 with big pockets and deep pleats. The larger sketch above is all about brisk plaid, for Spring 1967. Both show De De Johnson's look of quality casual.

victions. Understated, beautifully articulated, her fashions are of today, for the woman who loves quality."

Johnson introduced many fashion firsts over the course of her long career. In 1944, it was the pedal pusher; in 1946, it was culottes, which she dubbed the *Cloud Stroller*. She's credited with discovering the synthetic doeskin Caresseude in 1949, presaging the popularity of Ultrasuede more than a decade later. Her creation of a band-top skirt in 1960 helped bring the dirndl into fashion, as an aspect of peasant dressing.

Irene Kasmer

More casual clothing innovations came from Irene Kasmer, who immigrated to Los Angeles as a teenager in 1948. She soon found a job in the area's burgeoning garment industry. By 1958, she had created (and patented) the first Hip-Hugger pants. She derived the name from the obvious fact that these pants fell from the hip, not the waist, and from the emerging "hip" generation.

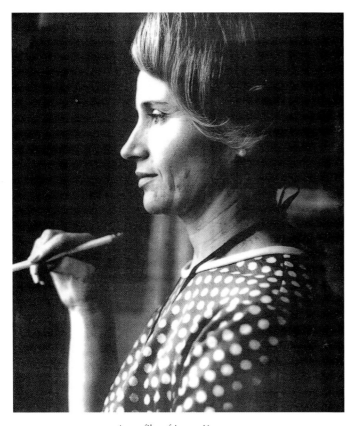

A profile of Irene Kasmer.

THE BIG SLEEVE

Fashion's preoccupation with details sometimes makes the big news story of the season. This spring it's the sudden emphasis on sleeves. We suspect it's a spin-off from recent romantic movies—*Romeo and Juliet, Elvira Madigan, Isadora*—but whatever the reason, billowing sleeves take over the spring scene. The fabrics keep pace with the soft silhouette and on this page Irene Kasmer has chosen strawberry-embroidered Dacron dotted swiss for the most romantic Juliet sleeve in the world. Its great fullness is caught in at the elbow and wrist in tiny gathers, and a ruffle completely covers the fingertips. At the Nobby Shops. At the top of the facing page is a giant red, white and blue print by DellaRossa Boutique, with sleeves that balloon out in the happy peasant influence. At the Apropos Stores. The huge organza sleeve, center right, springs out from a lowered shoulder line of heavy cotton lace and ends in a lace cuff. This is Travilla's fashion statement for spring in one of his most romantic moods in years. At Amelia Gray. The sleeve at lower right is a swoosh of silk-like acetate in a black and white abstract print. This is also by Irene Kasmer, who has again exaggerated the ruffle to cover the fingertips. At Joseph Magnin. The hair styles are by Hugh York, Saks Fifth Avenue.

Produced by Violet Weber
Photography: Mindas

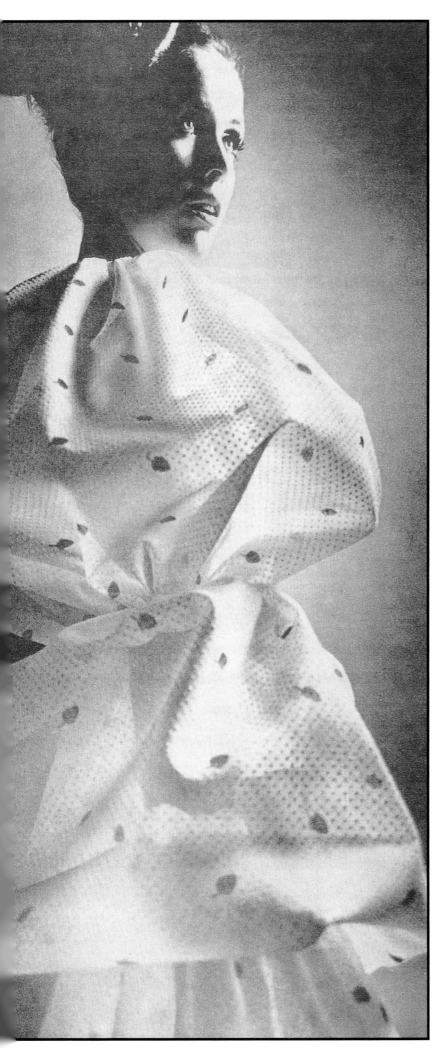

Like many who design in the casual genre, Kasmer was strongly inspired by new developments in fabric. She used Cone Fabrics' broad and pinwale corduroys extensively. She was also associated with Monsanto and is, in fact, credited with designing costumes for the audio-animatronic characters in Monsanto's *House of Tomorrow* exhibit at Disneyland.

Kasmer always promoted the California garment industry, and proudly labeled her garments "Irene Kasmer, Inc., California." Still active today from her offices in the Los Angeles Fashion Mart, she is seeking to find permanent quarters for her brainchild, the Museum of Fashion Designers and Creators. The museum will feature her own extensive collection of vintage California clothing.

Kasmer's billowing blouse made fashion news in the *Los Angeles Times* of February 1962, with focus on the fabric:

"Fashion's preoccupation with details . . . This season it's the sudden emphasis on sleeves . . . The fabrics keep pace with the soft silhouette and on this page Irene Kasmer has chosen strawberry-embroidered Dacron cotton swiss for the most romantic Juliet sleeve in the world. Its great fullness is caught in at the elbow and wrist in tiny gathers, and a ruffle completely covers the fingertips."

That's a big sleeve!

Addie Masters

Addie Masters had a keen eye for the type of clothing that a woman of wealth and taste wanted for "little evenings" with reference to the new pants silhouette. (In the early 1920s, Parisiennes had been mad for the silken lounging pajamas designed by Paul Poiret. In the late 1930s, women all over the world craved the exotic harem pants designed by Adrian for Jean Harlow in *Mata Hari*.)

Masters began her career in 1940, and had immediate success with a line of hostess pajamas with voluminous legs, combining the grace of a skirt and the ease of pants. Her self-stated objective was to design lovely at-home clothes, based on her belief that women are most beautiful in their own homes.

Masters infused patio dressing with the rich, sunny colors of California. Her full-cut palazzo pants had the pizzazz of bright floral prints, and her lightweight jersey gowns glowed in colors like lime, azure, and terra cotta. Deviating slightly from her pool and patio pathway, Masters designed little daytimers in sunny shades of cotton, sharkskin, and rayon. She was also famous for the *Wrap Rascal*. This casual slip-on dress preceded the Diane Von Furstenburg wrap by over a decade.

sun goddess

To glorify a girl, to make a goddess of you . . Addie Masters takes colors out of the sun, contrasts them boldly: fiery-red with lime or dazzling white; royal blue with lime or white . . two-color drama achieved by diamond inserts, crushed cummerbund. Patio dress for a lovely loafer, for a hostess . . in cool Celanese jersey.

Fred Matthews

A sophisticated gown for little evenings at home, featured in the *California Stylist* of April 1948. This patiogoer was cut from Celanese jersey in paprika or azure blue, mixed with lime or white.

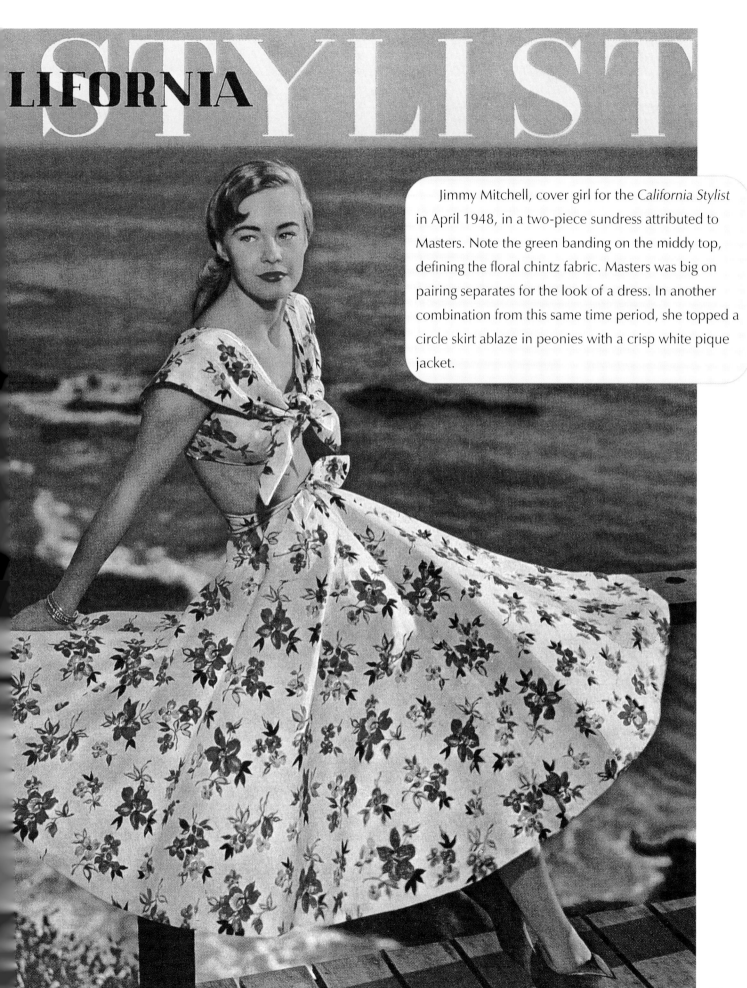

CALIFORNIA STYLIST

Jimmy Mitchell, cover girl for the *California Stylist* in April 1948, in a two-piece sundress attributed to Masters. Note the green banding on the middy top, defining the floral chintz fabric. Masters was big on pairing separates for the look of a dress. In another combination from this same time period, she topped a circle skirt ablaze in peonies with a crisp white pique jacket.

Pat Premo

Pat Premo was born and raised in the small California town of Porterville, from where she was motivated to find her future in fashion. Having moved to Los Angeles, she began working for Peggy Hunt in the early 1930s and joined the Marjorie Montgomery firm in 1936.

When entrepreneur Bill Schminke bought the firm a few years later, love and business blossomed. He married Pat, moved their headquarters, and opened W.J. Schminke & Associates with "Pat Premo" as the chief label. It was the beginning of what the *California Stylist* called a family dynasty, reflecting full involvement by their son, Bob Schminke.

"Pat Premo designs in the true California tradition," the *Stylist* boasted in a feature story of February 1968. "Like many lady-designers, her success has been based on the fact that she designs the kind of clothes that she and her friends like to wear."

Pat Premo produced frocks that could be dressed up or down. This one, in cool white cotton with exaggerated eyelet for the bodice, was advertised in Spring 1956.

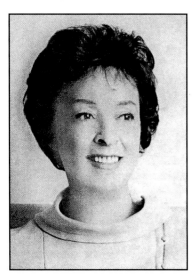

Pat Premo.

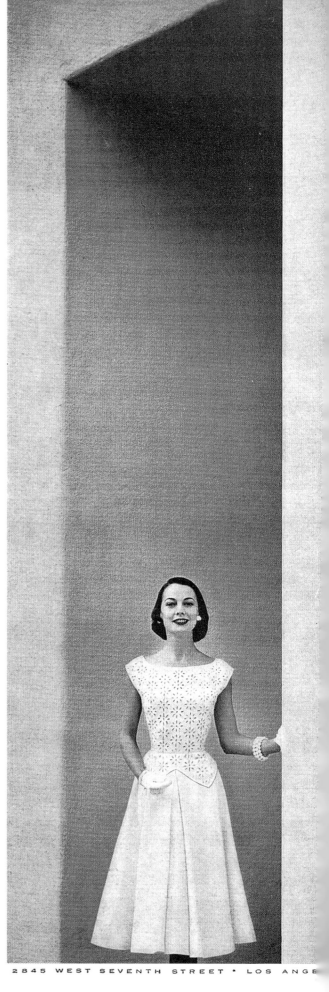

2845 WEST SEVENTH STREET · LOS ANGE

remo's line started with *Fireside Fashions* and important little dresses for late-day. As she developed an interest in golfing, it expanded into sportier clothes and golf dresses. In the mid-1960s, she created a *Suburbanite* group of casual styles for active women. In every collection, Premo placed great emphasis on quality fabrics, and often custom-ordered unique prints or colors to achieve the desired effect.

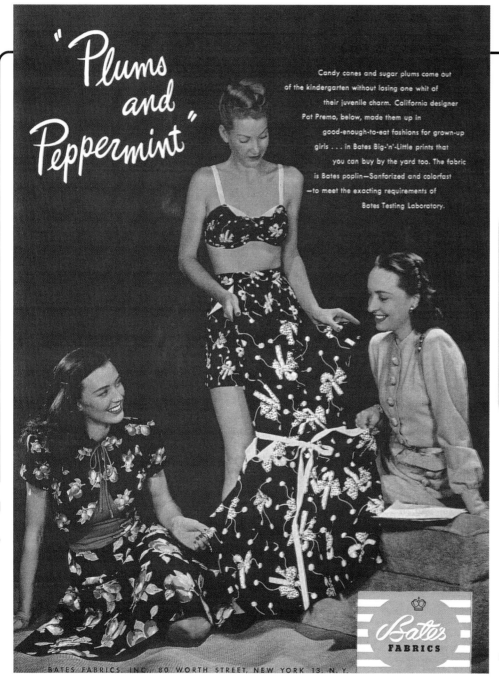

"Plums and Peppermint"

Candy canes and sugar plums come out of the kindergarten without losing one whit of their juvenile charm. California designer Pat Premo, below, made them up in good-enough-to-eat fashions for grown-up girls . . . in Bates Big-'n'-Little prints that you can buy by the yard too. The fabric is Bates poplin—Sanforized and colorfast —to meet the exacting requirements of Bates Testing Laboratory.

Bates
FABRICS

BATES FABRICS, INC., 80 WORTH STREET, NEW YORK 13, N. Y.

When Pat Premo chose these printed poplins in the Spring of 1946, she was promoted by Bates Fabrics in a national ad campaign. Both patterns were sold by the yard in "big 'n little" prints. (The bow-tied candy canes are amusing, for resortwear.)

Plums and Peppermint for 1946.

Joy Stevens

Joy Stevens was a girl wonder of the garment industry, having joined her father's firm as a designer at the age of seventeen. In this case, it may have been prophetic that dad named his Los Angeles business "Joy Stevens" in honor of his baby daughter.

Operating at first on borrowed capital, with a closet-size office and a shared contractor, Ben Stevens built his business on one blouse style: a pin-tucked Gibson Girl revival that wholesaled for $2.50 in the early 1940s. In 1957, he was doing $3 million a year from what is known in the trade as a "blouse house."

When Joy joined the firm in 1963, she shook it up with the bold new styles that her generation would want to wear. Ben might protest that they were too far-out, but she was adamant: "But, Daddy! This is fashion. We're in the *fashion* business!"

Young Joy Stevens often modeled her own line, as seen in this ad from May 1969.

JOY STEVEN

CREATES EXOTIC FASHION DRAMA IN PRINTS WITH THE ROMANTIC MYST

JOY STEVENS • NEW YORK, 1407 BROADWAY
DALLAS, DALLAS APPAREL MART RM. 2014 • MIAMI,

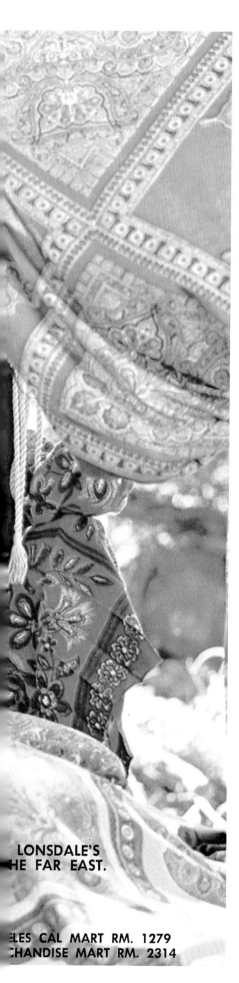

Sensitive to trends, but well-schooled in the most technical aspects of the business, Joy explained her philosophy to the *California Stylist* in 1967: "Fashion, as I see it, is a constant revolution dedicated to the young, not just the chronologically young, but those personalities that are active and aware of the time's development.

"We are dressing the woman literally from head to toe, accessorizing the garment with watches, headwear, bags, and everything else which can help today's woman find her fashion look in one convenient location."

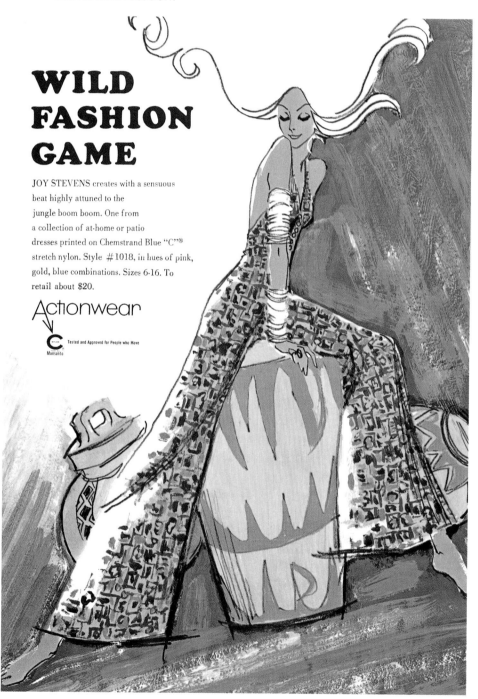

WILD FASHION GAME

JOY STEVENS creates with a sensuous beat highly attuned to the jungle boom boom. One from a collection of at-home or patio dresses printed on Chemstrand Blue "C"® stretch nylon. Style #1018, in hues of pink, gold, blue combinations. Sizes 6-16. To retail about $20.

Actionwear

C
Monsanto
Tested and Approved for People who Move

Joy's bold credo was reflected in this design for a wild jumpsuit with an African beat, as advertised in January 1967.

Elza of Hollywood

Many of the artisans profiled here could not have done their pioneering work without the fine fabrics of Elza Sunderland. In the 1940s and 1950s, she designed more than two thousand patterns for her own firm, Elza of Hollywood. For a 1986 retrospective of her work at the Los Angeles County Museum of Art, curator Edward Maeder reflected on the impact she had on daily life across America: "[Elza] changed the way people dressed and decorated their homes, helping to institute the use of new fabrics, colors and styles—all part of the 'California look'."

Sunderland opened shop in 1937, at a time when all things Californian were in fashion. It seemed as if the nation could not get enough of the happy, healthy relaxed styles that were considered natural attributes of life in this sunshine state. For many designers, including Sunderland, it was not only a question of talent—but of being in the right place, at the right time.

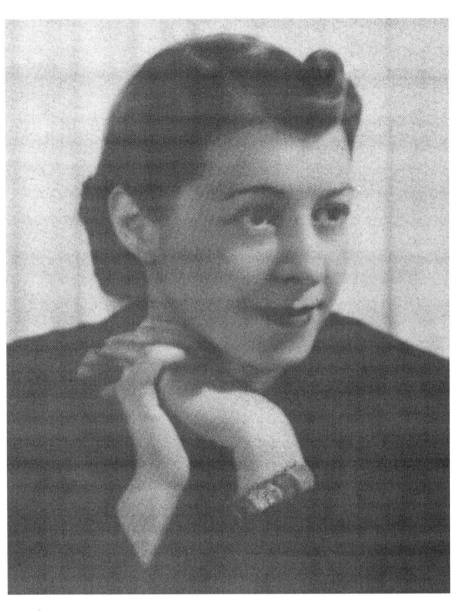

Elza Sunderland, 1939.

"In Elza's time there was a new demand for practical casual dress for shopping, for patio entertaining, beach outings, and tennis. Swimwear was 'big' and for the first time printed patterns were being used for bathing suits," wrote Maeder. "New fabrics were being used for these lightweight garments. In the midst of World War II it was difficult, if not impossible, to obtain textiles such as wool and silk from the traditional centers of production in Europe and the Far East. Advances in textile technology brought new 'wonder fabrics' such as spun rayon and acetates. They were declared superior to many of the natural fibers in nationwide advertising campaigns. The California climate was well-suited for these lightweight fabrics, and the California fashion designers were open to using them."

Opposite page
The roaming *Strawberry* pattern was inspired by abundant plants growing in the backyard of Sunderland's own home in Los Angeles.

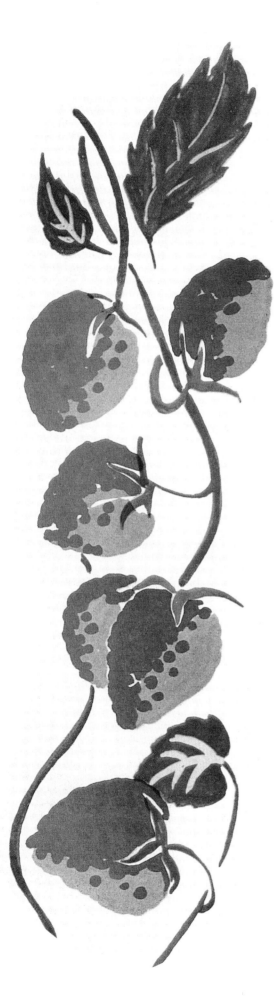

Perhaps it's only fitting that Sunderland, like so many other success stories, came to this young state as an immigrant from old Europe. The six-year-old Elza Wilheim arrived in New York City in 1910, with the rest of her artistic family. (Her mother took the children on museum outings; her two brothers became fine art painters). She studied design and took textile courses at Washington Irving High School, which specialized in the arts. Upon graduation she landed her first job hand-painting lampshades for a studio in Brooklyn.

In 1923, upon her marriage to Dan Sunderland, she took a career hiatus to be a full-time wife and homemaker. Their son Henry was born in 1929. But the creative juices were still flowing, and when the Sunderlands moved to Los Angeles in 1937, she set up shop. As she stated in a 1948 magazine interview, California was "the dream" that she could only hope to capture in textiles. It was a land lush with foliage, fruit, and ripe opportunity.

Sunderland rendered the Western landscape, with its native plants and animals, into textile designs of great originality. Her fabric names speak volumes: *Desert Flower, Blooming Cactus, Monterey Rose, Fiesta,* and *Gold Rush*. While these prints could be custom-ordered in bulk, they were also sold off-the-bolt to the average homemaker and her daughter.

With the home market in mind, Sunderland carefully placed her pattern repeats so they could be readily measured and cut by a novice seamstress. As explained in a magazine feature of 1948: "[The] pattern was put on the material in such a way that it might be cut variously without disturbing the print in the least, making it easy for the beginner to visualize . . . one of Elza's 'make life easier' ideas in fabric."

Perhaps Sunderland's most popular pattern was *Strawberry*, a vivid spray of mouth-watering fruit designed as a border. After its release in 1943, the cheerful pattern remained popular for over a decade. It was typically translated into kitchen curtains, napkins, and tablecloths. More than 250,000 yards were eventually sold in fabric stores across the nation, a true tribute to Sunderland's goal of helping women make attractive homes.

While most designers would create their own patterns, Sunderland was one of the few who could personally convert them from paper to finished product. By dint of her technical assurance, Sunderland saw the potential for producing printed rayon, acetate, and Lastex. She was also an innovator with natural fibers like cotton, and was the first to design printed terrycloth.

Her fresh fabrics were a natural medium for designers in the emerging sportswear industry. Sunderland began working with the designers almost immediately upon opening her own company, and continued this relationship until her retirement in 1955. As one of the first textile designers to understand the potential of the elasticized "miracle fibers" that were so vital to swimwear, she worked with Margit Felligi for Cole, Mary Ann DeWeese for Catalina, and Rose Marie Reid.

Sunderland's design range was vast, enabling her to realize her "dream" of California in versatile fabrics that were suitable for commercial or home use. She also brought the recognition of quality goods to a middle-class market, with steady emphasis on value and suitability. "I think a woman who pays a dollar a yard deserves as much consideration as the one paying five dollars," she once explained, "and my inexpensive prints are created with that thought in mind."

Sunderland, the immigrant egalitarian who brought elegance into everywoman's home, donated her entire collection of textile samples and sketches to the Los Angeles County Museum of Art in 1985.

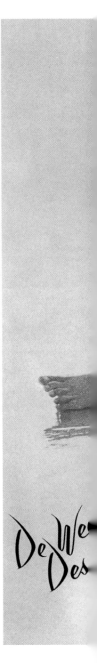

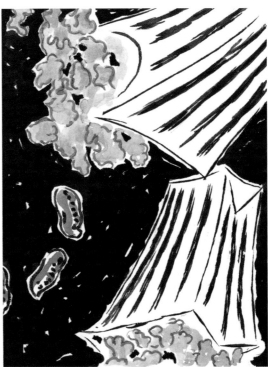

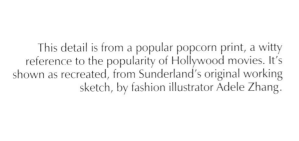

This detail is from a popular popcorn print, a witty reference to the popularity of Hollywood movies. It's shown as recreated, from Sunderland's original working sketch, by fashion illustrator Adele Zhang.

chapter 2

ON THE BEACH

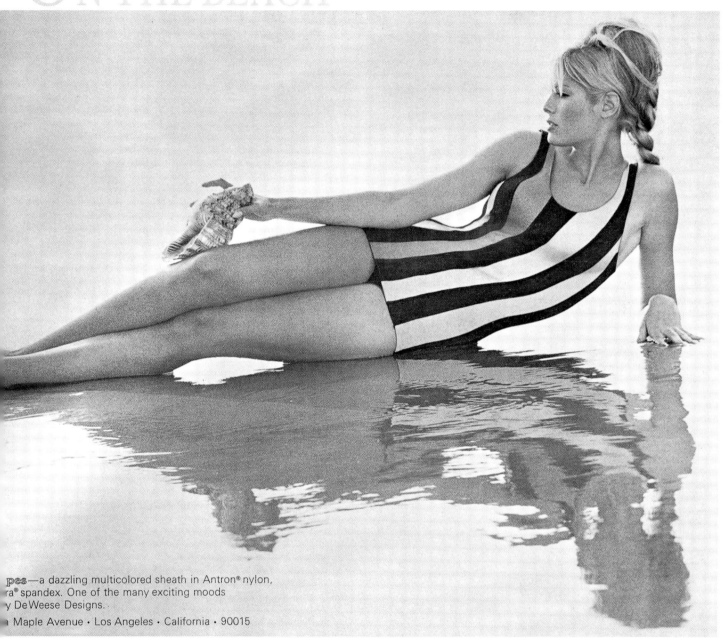

pes—a dazzling multicolored sheath in Antron® nylon,
ra® spandex. One of the many exciting moods
y DeWeese Designs.

Maple Avenue · Los Angeles · California · 90015

A streamlined, functional suit advertised by DeWeese in October 1967.

"The history of the American swimsuit is the square-inch-by-square-inch story of how skin went public in modern times. In an equally important sense, it is also the story of how flesh and fabric have come together to serve sport, sex, and culture."

—Lena Lencek and Gideon Bosker, *Making Waves*, 1989.

We've come a long way baby. From black serge bloomer suits in 1901, to the Topless in 1964; thence to the Thong in 1979. The saga of swimwear is shaped by a tug-of-war between conventional mores pulling for modesty on one side, and basic instincts wrenching toward exposure on the other. As we all know, exposure won out.

So what's left to come off, up, or down in the year 2001? The business of predicting fashion trends is tricky at best. It's nearly impossible when form must follow function, as with swimwear. That's not to say the fashion press doesn't try.

In late 1999, asked to make a new-millennium fashion prediction by the *Los Angeles Times*, Anne Cole drawled: "Bikini, tankini, what does it matter daaarling . . . so long as you're sipping a maaartini." An amusing and telling observation, from the scion of a swimwear company that was famous for glamorous and sophisticated designs.

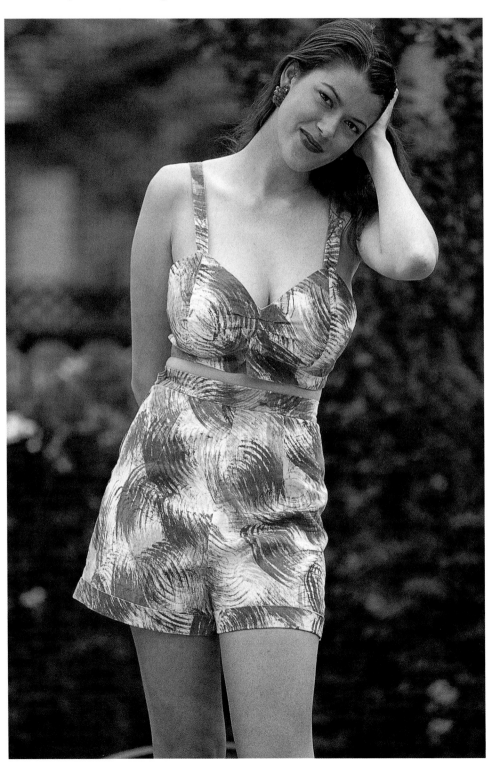

A peek at what was daring circa 1945, when actress Dorothy Lamour popularized tropical prints. Here, barkcloth print shorts complement a halter top (no label) on Chrystal Williams . Value: $55-75. *Courtesy, Luxe.*

The Swimwear Alliance That Almost Was

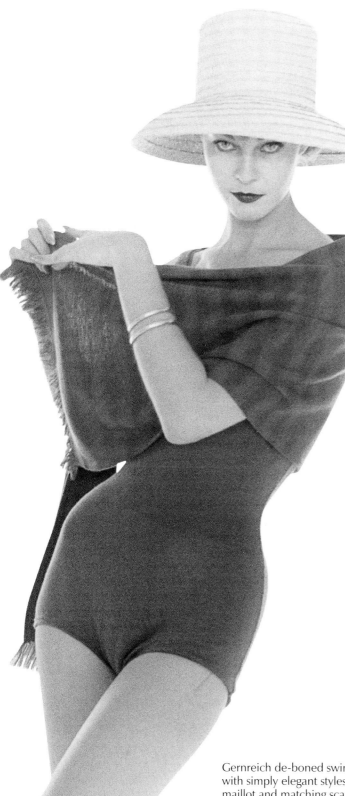

Gernreich de-boned swimsuits in the 1950s,
with simply elegant styles like this knit
maillot and matching scarf.

Fashion changes in some way every season, even every six months," Anne Cole recently observed. "Eventually, the fashion cycle is identified with a particular designer, or generation." Given her understanding of this pattern, it is one of the industry's little-known ironies that she discouraged Rudi Gernreich from working as a free-lance designer for her father.

"It was in early 1960, when my father made his first trip to Tahiti, and he arranged to put Rudi in charge of the collection for the coming season. Now, I knew Rudi was brilliant, but I also knew it was because he was defying *conventional* fashion. His swimwear was clean and simple. I was afraid we'd ruin him! I mean, he'd lose his design eye if he had to turn out *structured* suits, the type we were selling."

She knew whereof she spoke. One of Anne Cole's favorite sales tips was a reminder to size up the customer's figure type with reference to structure: "Think of the bra as a two-car garage; if you have a little sports car to park, why that's fine; if you have a Cadillac, so much the better."

Women's and men's swimsuits had evolved into the classic maillot by the mid-1920s, with little design distinction made for gender. Ten years later, men were finally wearing the two-piece suit, sometimes with a zippered waistline that allowed them to remove the top half. Still, they were risking arrest on a public beach!

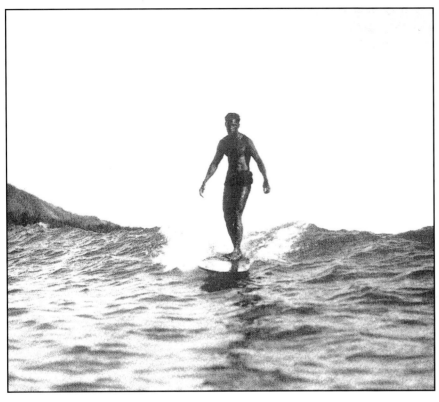

Hawaiian surfing champion Duke Kahanamoku wore a *Wicki* one-piecer in the summer of 1929. *Courtesy, Library of Congress.*

In the 1920s, a younger generation of sports-minded Gantners joined the venerable Gantner-Mattern Co. of San Francisco. One of them visited Hawaii and was taken with the island sport of surfing, performed by young men who dared to bare their chests on the beach. This brought the topless *Wicki* suit into production, so named because surfing spectators in Hawaii would urge on their favorite athletes with cries of "wicki" or "hurry up." The trunks were knitted with a patented high waist, and the Hawaiian surfing champions became the first converts.

Two-piece suits for women made their first appearance in the mid-1940s, typically with a sarong bottom and a halter top. Some suits from this era featured a midriff cutout, for the sexiness of a two-piece with the security of a maillot. The strapless maillot made a big splash in the 1950s—in keeping with a craze for the same style in formal gowns.

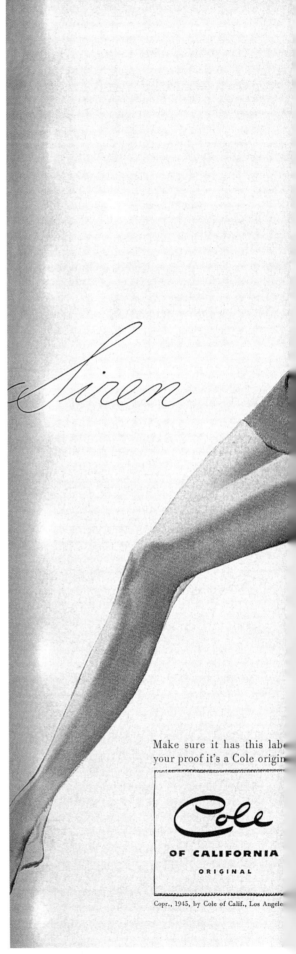

Siren

Make sure it has this label your proof it's a Cole original

Cole
OF CALIFORNIA
ORIGINAL

Copr., 1945, by Cole of Calif., Los Angeles

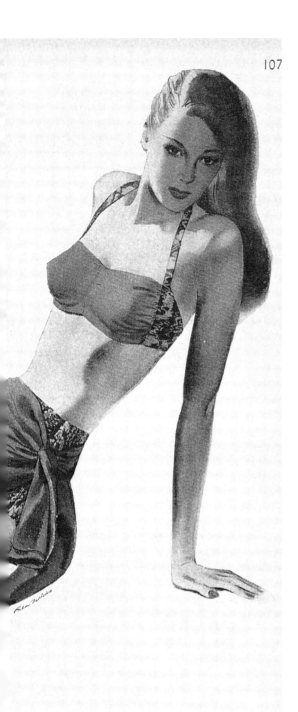

107

Two-piece suits got skimpier until the bikini bombshell dropped at a poolside fashion show in Paris on July 5, 1946. The creation of French couturier Jacques Heim, it was originally dubbed the "atome." But it was such a style explosion, the world press adopted an even more provocative name, coined by rival designer Louis Reard. He named it "bikini," after the Pacific Ocean atoll where the U.S. government was then testing Atom bombs.

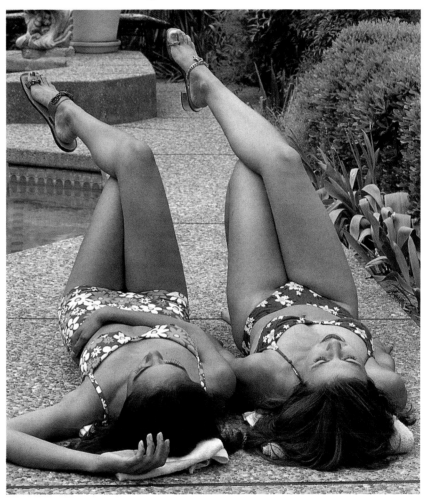

The bikini was emblematic of Sexy Sixties fashions.

This sarong-styled two-piece, the *Siren Suit* by Cole, was advertised in November 1945.

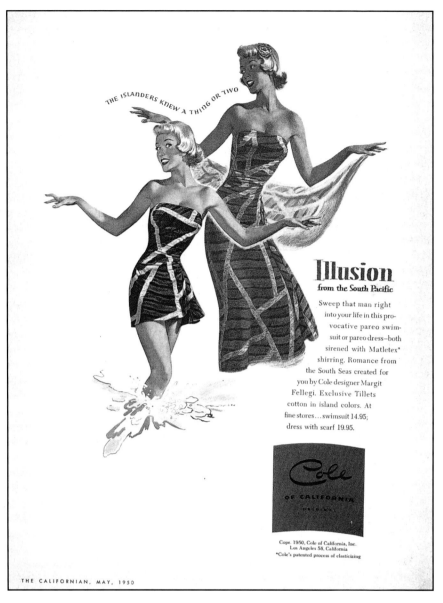

A coordinated sundress might be offered in lieu of a cover-up. This duet was advertised in May 1950: "[A] provocative pareo . . . sirened with Matletex © shirring. Romance from the South Seas created for you by Cole designer Margit Felligi." The cost was $14.95 (swimsuit) or $19.95 (dress/scarf).

The bikini was an immediate sensation at Cannes and other French resorts, but the more conservative American public would not accept the daring new style for more than a decade. Remember the *Itsy Bitsy, Teeny Weeny, Yellow Polka-Dot Bikini* ditty? It was released by Brian Hyland in 1960.

All these brief new styles required cover-ups, and manufacturers were quick to establish a market for coordinated beach coats, pajama pants, pirate shorts, wrap skirts, and pareos.

The swimwear industry originated on the West Coast in the 1920s with three big firms, all of which had morphed from knitwear. Jantzen was originally the Portland Knitting Mills; Cole was West Coast Knitting Mills; and Catalina was Bentz Knitting Mills. Moreover, they were all inspired by the glamour of early Hollywood. It was a natural liaison, given the proliferation of publicity shots showing starlets in skimpy bathing suits.

Opposite page
Esther Williams in her namesake suit by Cole of California. The star, and her sync swim chorus, were decked out in Cole for *Neptune's Daughter (1949)*, *Skirts Ahoy (1952)*, and *Dangerous When Wet (1953)*.

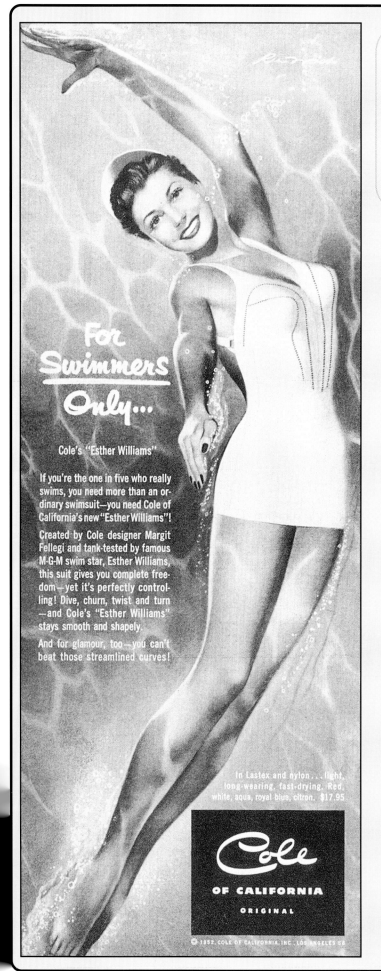

For Swimmers Only...

Cole's "Esther Williams"

If you're the one in five who really swims, you need more than an ordinary swimsuit—you need Cole of California's new "Esther Williams"!

Created by Cole designer Margit Fellegi and tank-tested by famous M-G-M swim star, Esther Williams, this suit gives you complete freedom—yet it's perfectly controlling! Dive, churn, twist and turn —and Cole's "Esther Williams" stays smooth and shapely.

And for glamour, too—you can't beat those streamlined curves!

In Lastex and nylon... light, long-wearing, fast-drying. Red, white, aqua, royal blue, citron. $17.95

Cole
OF CALIFORNIA
ORIGINAL

© 1952, COLE OF CALIFORNIA, INC., LOS ANGELES 58

Fred Cole contracted with Esther Williams to promote his bathing suits in advertisements like this one from 1952. The Lastex-and-nylon *Esther Williams* suit hugged every curve. Its top-stitched *ballet bodice* was "tank tested" by Williams. Cole hoped to get screen credits for other suits worn by Williams in a variety of movies, but MGM was not forthcoming.

S wimwear manufacturers recruited fashion designers like Louella
Ballerino, who created an ethnic collection for Jantzen in the
1940s, and Emilio Pucci, who made color-block ponchos for Rose
Marie Reid in the 1950s.

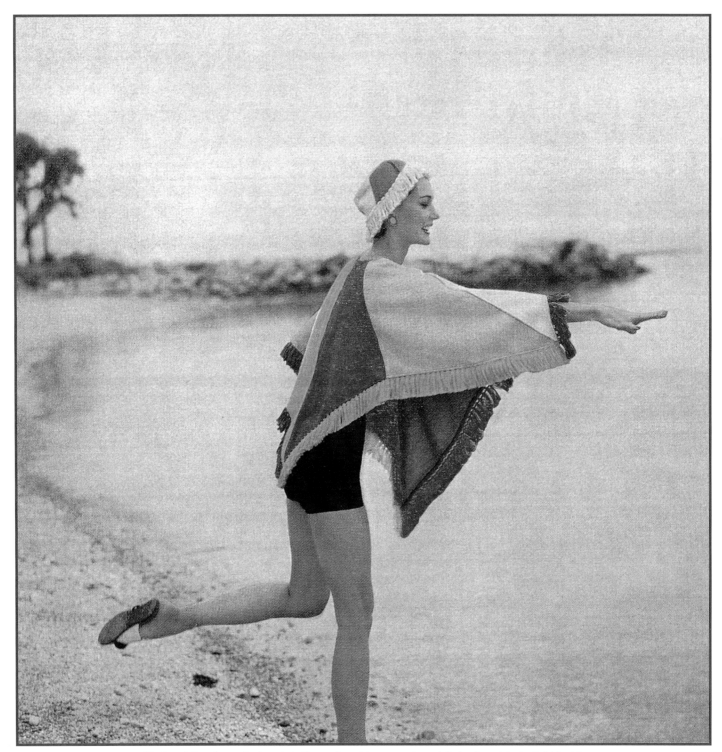

Emilio Pucci free-lanced a beach-ball poncho with cap and sandals for Rose Marie Reid in 1955.

The biggest contributing factor in the development of swimwear lay not in artistry, but in science: the discovery of Lastex in the early 1930s. This was an elasticized fiber that shed water and retained its shape; better yet, it *reined in* shape.

The stretchy fabric acted like a girdle, molding the average woman's wayward figure. Manufacturers were quick to capitalize on this feature with built-in boning, bra cups, and other traditional aspects of corseting. In the mid-1930s, Cole's head designer Margit Felligi took the idea a step further with her patented *Matletex* process that warp-knit a rigid fabric like cotton with elastic thread, to create a flattering shirred effect. Rose Marie Reid also used Lastex to great advantage.

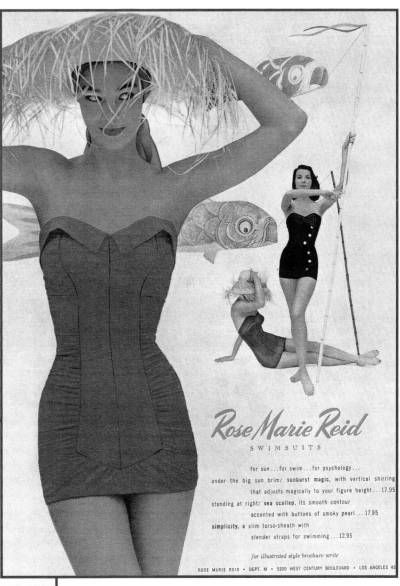

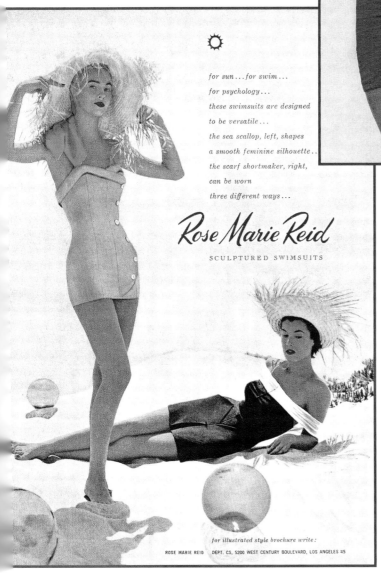

Hot in pink, the *Sunburst Magic* maillot with all the structure of a ballgown. Advertised by Rose Marie Reid in 1951 as part of a shirred and tucked group cut from figure-controlling Lastex.

The most elastic miracle fabric of all was Spandex, a synthetic polyurethane that became generally available in the early 1960s. It consisted of a foam core that could be covered with silk, cotton, wool, or other natural fibers to make a stretchy, lightweight yarn. Spandex (or Lycra, the trade name patented by DuPont) was stretchable and lightweight, yet possessed enough tension to provide the best figure control available in swimwear.

The experiments continued until 1964, when Felligi commissioned another special fiber for Cole. It was Spandex with a twist, since natural fiber was wrapped around a foam core in a spiral pattern, then shaped into a fishnet mesh with enough tension to pull expanses of bare skin into taut shape. Tension, skin, and sex were all it took to make the *Scandal Suit* one of the biggest sellers in the history of sportswear.

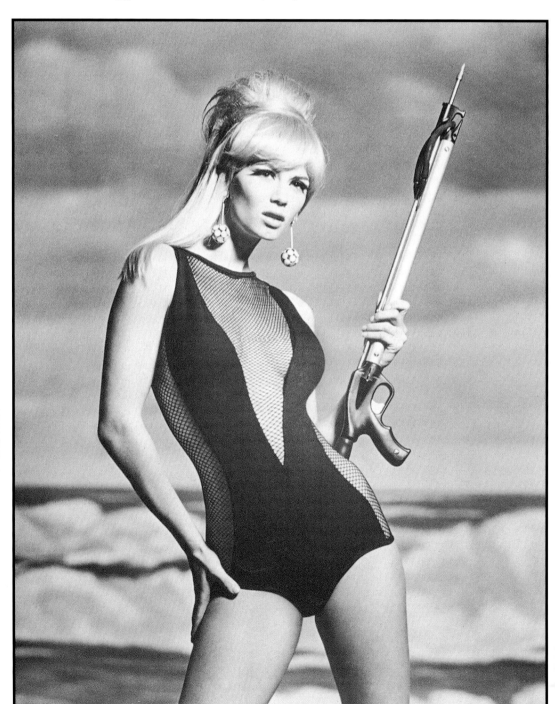

The *Scandal Suit* as featured on page one of the *Wall Street Journal* in 1965. Its taut netting created tension on the beach and cast newspaper headlines.

Like other casual clothing, vintage swimwear is sometimes difficult to locate —it was worn so frequently as to be worn out. Still, there are occasional finds of "dead stock" suits along with beach cover-ups, and those amusing flowered bathing caps. Given that the industry is closely aligned with new fabric technologies, this is a rewarding specialty area for the vintage collector.

That Stretchy Jantzen Stitch

In 1920, a ribbed-knit rowing outfit was adapted to swimwear for athletic competition by Carl Jantzen of Portland, Oregon. His business, which was to become a swimwear empire, was based on this new technology whereby knitting machines acted in tandem. Using the classic rib stitch, each set worked at right angles to the other: one pulled the stitch out from one side of the fabric, the other pulled ribbing from the alternate side. The result was a knit with twice the elasticity of wool jersey, ideal for athletic competition.

Jantzen is often mistaken for a California company, perhaps due to the fact that Hollywood stars like Loretta Young, Marilyn Monroe, and Rita Hayworth were featured in ad campaigns. More likely, the mix-up stems from Jantzen's proximity to the endless summer coastline of California.

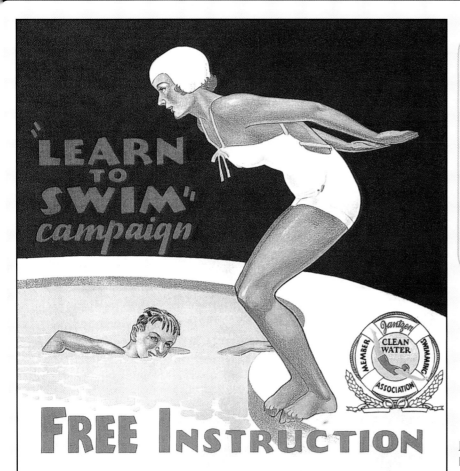

With partners John and Roy Zehntbauer, owners of the Portland Knitting Company, Carl Jantzen built a sportswear empire based on his invention of the right-angled elastic stitch. Since beginning operations in 1921, Jantzen has styled suits for active swimmers, with a red-suited girl diver as logo. To build its market, the company promoted athletic competition.

Jantzen launched a national Learn to Swim campaign in 1926, as a means of boosting sales.

Cole of California

For decades, swimwear has dipped into the creative waters of movie costume design. It started in the early 1920s when Fred Cole, a silent film actor, persuaded his parents to start a swimwear line at their knitting mills in Los Angeles. His task was made easier by the fact that his mother thought *acting* was hardly a respectable career for her son.

Cole's parents, Edith and Morris Cohn, were themselves the children of garment manufacturers. They were both born into pioneering blue jean companies in California—notably the Boss label on the side of his grandfather Cohn (who later changed his name to Cole). Cole's parents formed the West Coast Manchester Knitting Mills—from blue denim to pool blue, as it were. Their son officially opened the mill's swimwear division on May 15, 1925. The original line of socks and longjohns quickly diminished in favor of swimwear production, until Fred Cole discarded the voluminous name of his parent's knitting mill in favor of "Cole of California"—a name change recorded on January 15, 1941.

In launching the mill's new line, it was only natural that the former actor and self-styled playboy would turn to the bathing beauty look then being launched in Hollywood. It was a concept that met with instant approval in the marketplace, leading Cole to scout for full-fledged Hollywood design talent. He found it in Margit Felligi, who would rule as the company's head designer from 1936 through 1972.

Felligi's reign was one of spectacular innovation, especially in the use of fabric. In the first year of her hire, she retrofit old knitting machines to produce the patented *Matletex* process that shirred any natural fiber, primarily cotton, by warp-knitting it with a rubber-based Lastex thread.

In 1943, to compensate for the wartime shortage of rubber, Felligi created the first side-laced swimsuit. Dubbed the *Swoon Suit* in honor of the young crooner Frank Sinatra, it was made in one- and two-piece styles from the same silk Cole was stitching into parachutes.

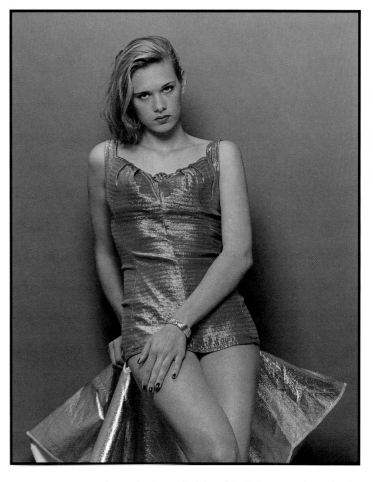

An early glam suit (pin added), in turquoise veined with 24K gold thread. Margit Felligi incorporated luxury fabrics like this, in designs for Cole of California.

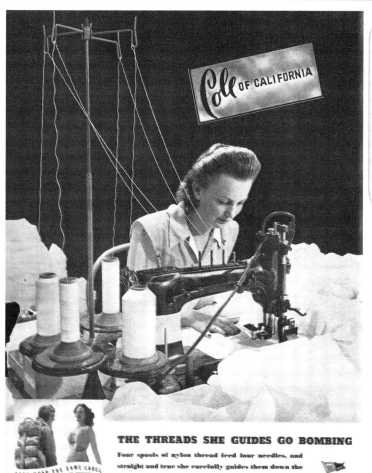

Fred Cole was awarded a government contract to produce parachutes due to the expertise of his production crew and, in part, to the extra-long cutting tables in his factory. During the war years, Felligi continued to design a limited number of suits to keep the Cole label alive, produced in a small plant that she opened for that purpose in Santa Barbara.

Cole was proud of its role in the war, when the knitting mill was used as a parachute factory. This January 1944 ad explains how four spools of nylon thread feed four needles to work the silk. "The Threads She Guides Go Bombing."

THE THREADS SHE GUIDES GO BOMBING

Four spools of nylon thread feed four needles, and straight and true she carefully guides them down the long mainseams of a parachute canopy. She excelled in peacetime making Cole Swim suits. Now her everyday skill has gained perfection—for a flyer's lifeline.

Keep asking—some Cole Swim suits are available at the better stores.

The *Swoon Suit* as advertised in January 1944. Its side lacing was not only sexy, it served to give fragile silk the figure-controlling characteristics of a rubber girdle. It was one of the few styles produced by Cole during the war years. "Today we give precedence to parachutes, make only a limited number of Cole swim and play fashions."

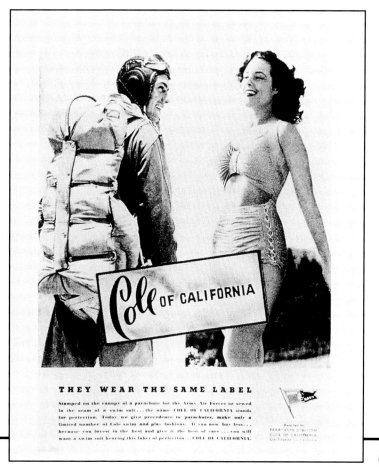

THEY WEAR THE SAME LABEL

Stamped on the canopy of a parachute for the Army Air Forces or sewed in the seam of a swim suit...the name COLE OF CALIFORNIA stands for perfection. Today we give precedence to parachutes, make only a limited number of Cole swim and play fashions. If you now buy less...because you invest in the best and give it the best of care...you will want a swim suit bearing this label of perfection...COLE OF CALIFORNIA.

dding to her firsts, Felligi used Helanca nylon for swimwear in 1954. Ten years later she twisted Spandex fibers to create the springy fishnet mesh behind her front-running "scandal" collection.

According to a tribute in the *California Stylist* of February 1967, this prolific designer must also be credited with a long list of style scoops: coordinated cover-ups, bared midriffs, side-swept draping, and the blouson top.

Not that Felligi's designs ever became too fantastic to function. "After all," she told the *Stylist*, "swimwear is worn at leisure time. It must be comfortable. It must make you feel good as well as look attractive. And it must look just as well from the back, otherwise you have just a strange wiggle-waggle."

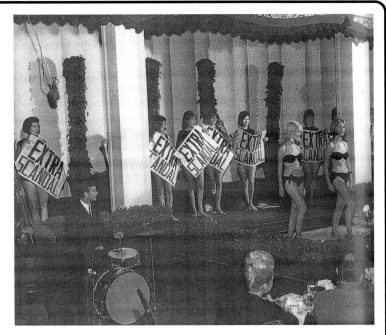

Scandalous headlines, with no wiggle-waggle.

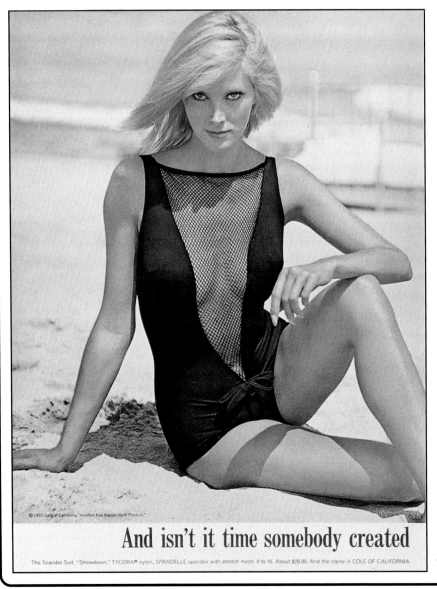

©1965 Cole of California. "Another fine Raymor-Roth Product."

And isn't it time somebody created

The Scandal Suit, "Showdown," TYCORA® nylon, SPANDELLE spandex with stretch mesh. 8 to 16. About $26.00. And the name is COLE OF CALIFORNIA.

The *Scandal Suit* was released to the fashion press in 1964, with a runway presentation of models holding mock front-page headlines screaming "scandal" in bold print. They dropped the papers on cue, revealing what was, at the time, one of the most overtly sexy and daring swimsuits ever marketed. According to Felligi, even nice girls would become a bit *scandalous* once they donned the sliced-up suit.

The *Scandal Suit* as advertised in 1965.

Felligi was born of Hungarian parentage in St. Louis, Missouri. She trained at the Chicago Academy of Fine Arts before making her debut as an *adagio* dancer in that city's famed Palace Theatre. The diminutive Felligi, who was just five feet tall and hovered at eighty-five pounds all her adult life, designed her own stage costumes. She soon gravitated to full-time design for the Keith-Orpheum theatre circuit. From there it was but a short trip to Hollywood.

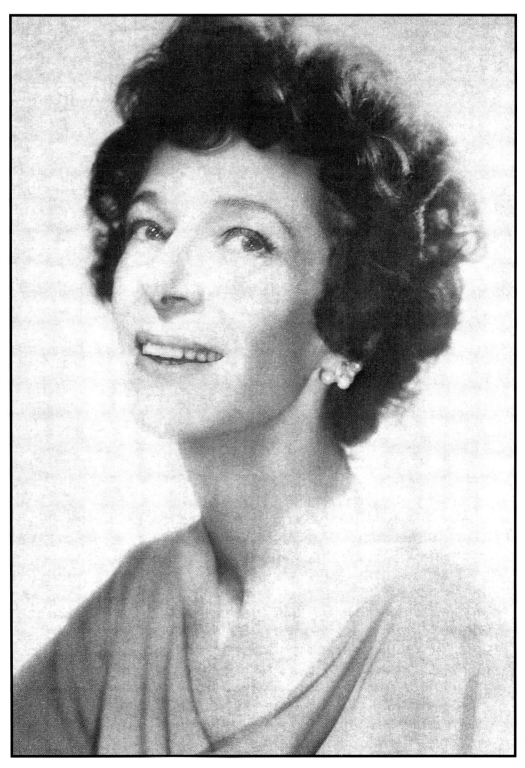

Margit Felligi, fabric maven.

Felligi moved to the upscale neighborhood of Beverly Hills, where her parents had already emigrated. She briefly opened a fashionable custom design studio, then worked as a free-lance costume designer—but her true calling became clear when she joined Cole in 1936.

This designer had an eye for the shock value of unusual fabrics that often seemed more suitable to the ballroom than the beach. She adapted luxury cloths like velvet and lamé, and discovered how to inset rhinestones so that they wouldn't degrade in the water.

She had a chance to test her high fashion instincts to the utmost in the mid-1950s, when Fred Cole exercised his flair for publicity by recruiting Christian Dior of Paris to design a special swimwear line. "As I recall," said Anne Cole, "Dior was reluctant because he didn't know anything about swimsuits. My father said, 'You're a designer aren't you? So, design.' Of course, Margit helped enormously in putting the collection together."

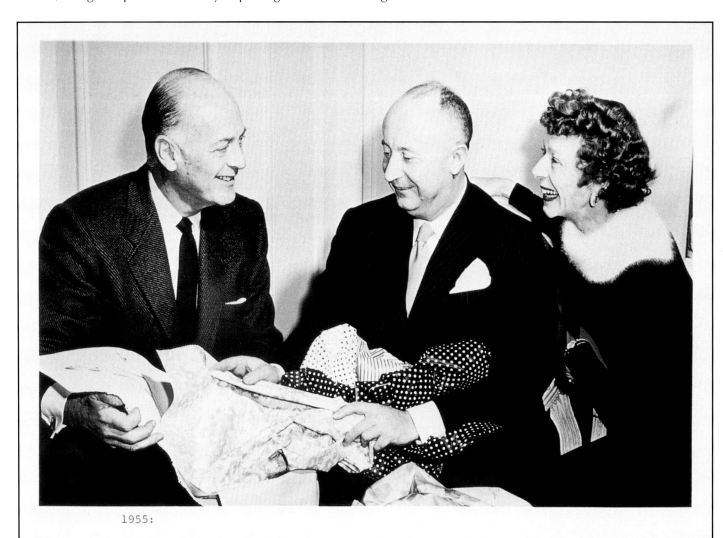

1955:

Left to right: Fred Cole, Christian Dior, and Margit Fellegi discussing fabric and design for the Cole-Dior Collection of 1955.

The Cole-Dior Collection debuted in 1955, just two years before the French designer's untimely death. In this photo from the Anne Cole Archives, Christian Dior (center) discusses fabric and design with Fred Cole and Margit Felligi.

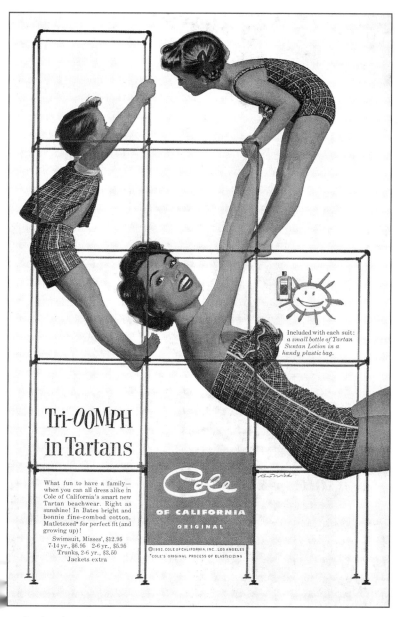

Tri-*OO*MPH
in Tartans

What fun to have a family—when you can all dress alike in Cole of California's smart new Tartan beachwear. Right as sunshine! In Bates bright and bonnie fine-combed cotton. Matletexed* for perfect fit (and growing up)!

Swimsuit, Misses', $12.95
7-14 yr., $6.95 2-6 yr., $5.95
Trunks, 2-6 yr., $3.50
Jackets extra

Included with each suit:
a small bottle of Tartan
Suntan Lotion in a
handy plastic bag.

Cole
OF CALIFORNIA
ORIGINAL

©1952, COLE OF CALIFORNIA, INC., LOS ANGELES
*COLE'S ORIGINAL PROCESS OF ELASTICIZING

The family is dressed for play in "smart new Tartan beachwear" in the Summer of 1951.

At the other end of the textile spectrum, Felligi stole sprightly prints from the nursery for rompers, grabbed terry toweling for bikinis, and played with plaid for mother-daughter duets. In the final analysis, she was nothing short of a technical genius, whose dazzling swimwear was constructed from the fiber right up to the furbelow.

Amusingly, her swim-spiration came only from the drawing board. Felligi was so diminutive, she refused to don her own designs. "Don't be silly, darling," she quipped. "I'd look like Mahatma Ghandi!"

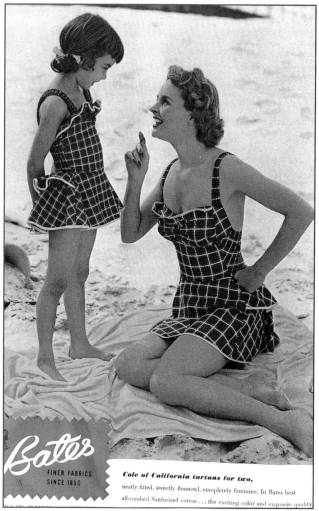

Bates
FINER FABRICS
SINCE 1850

Cole of California tartans for two,
neatly fitted, sweetly flounced, completely feminine. In Bates best all-combed Sanforized cotton . . . the exciting color and exquisite quality

Mother and daughter, tan and Tartan-ed.

When Fred Cole launched his swimwear line, he began a career marked as much by his own strong ego as by Felligi's design talent. Cole regularly hosted pool parties at his Beverly Hills home with models, whose role it was to display his latest lines *and* their lissome limbs.

On November 4, 1960, with an eye toward retirement, Cole sold the business outright to the hosiery manufacturer Kayser-Roth. He also sold a ten-year exclusive right to use the name "Cole of California." Felligi stayed on with the new company, as did many other staffers, so the sales beat didn't slow one bit.

Having raised a family of four with Alice, his wife of thirty years, the eccentric Fred decamped for Tahiti as soon as the ink was dry on the contract of sale. What began as a vacation transitioned into a stay of years, and divorce followed. He returned statewide shortly before his death, in 1964. (Ironically, that's the year his label received international publicity for the *Scandal Suit*.)

In his heyday during the Fab Fifties, Fred Cole was running an international multi-million-dollar corporation. This is when daughter Anne began to work for the company as a marketing representative. She quickly climbed the corporate ladder, and tells an amusing story about how she became a businesswoman role model.

"I got a phone call from an ad agency out of the blue, asking me to pose with a brand-new 1958 Thunderbird. They wanted to feature women at the wheel, or some such thing." The agency rep cajoled: "It will mean $1,000 to you." To which Cole replied: "Oh no! I don't have that kind of money!"

The mistake was quickly explained, and she appeared in national ads at the wheel of a convertible. The ad glowed: "The young and vivacious Vice-President of Cole of California commutes to her office (and cruises the country!) in her new Thunderbird."

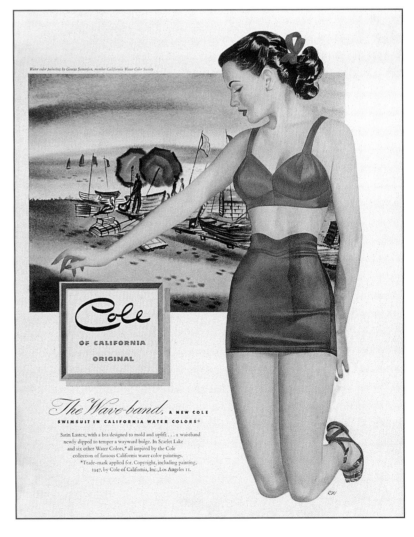

The Wave-band, as advertised by Cole of California in the late 1940s.

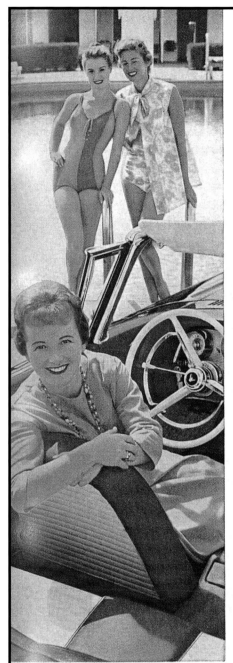

Anne Cole tells...

Why women love the new Thunderbird

The young and vivacious Vice-President of Cole of California commutes to her office (and crosses the country!) in her new Thunderbird

Anne Cole is one of the youngest, prettiest and most successful executives in the world of fashion. Her name and her swimsuits are known to fashion-conscious women all over the country. One of the rewards of success for Miss Cole is her new Thunderbird.

"It's a wonderful car," says Miss Cole. "When I'm in Los Angeles, I drive from my home to my office every day. It's only 20 miles—but you know L.A. traffic! Even so, I handle my T-bird as though I were the world's greatest driver, which I'm not. It's just that it's so easy to handle. It's so easy, in fact, that I drive from the Coast to New York twice a year. That's really traveling!

"What I mean is that other cars I've driven seem to have 'FOR MEN ONLY' signs on them. My Thunderbird says, 'ANNE COLE.' It's *my* car and I love it.

"My Thunderbird has flair!"

"It's a black convertible with a white top and it's beautiful. Personally, I think it's the smartest car on the road, with simple, classic understatement. If you don't like clutter, if you don't like busyness . . . you'll like the Thunderbird. But, as you know, I *do* like flair in design and the Thunderbird has great flair!

"The Thunderbird is so luxurious, too. Contoured seats add such a nice touch. They're wide and deep and couldn't be more comfortable. You don't feel as though you're sitting on the floor when you sit in a Thunderbird! And I like having the service console separating the seats. Very smart. And *practical*.

"I like the wide doors. No matter what I'm wearing, I can get in and out with no effort at all. A blessing!

"But do you know what I like best of all? The way I *look* in my Thunderbird! It makes me look *glamorous*. I *feel* glamorous in it. It's that kind of car. And let's face it—a car is an accessory these days. And accessories must be smart."

See how *you* look in a Thunderbird

Next time you look at cars with your husband, let him see how you look in a Thunderbird. Let him see how he *feel* in a Thunderbird. Let him drive it around the corner—just once will do it—and he'll buy it for you. You'll have a Thunderbird all your own!

Your Ford dealer invites you to compare luxury cars for beauty, comfort and glamour. Do this and you'll agree with Anne Cole that the new Thunderbird is "the smartest car on the road." Yet the 1959 Thunderbird costs *far* less than other luxury cars!

FORD DIVISION, *Ford Motor Company*

"My Thunderbird *fits me*," rejoices Miss Cole. "It's just my size. This makes so much difference in how you feel at the wheel. And how you handle yourself—and the car."

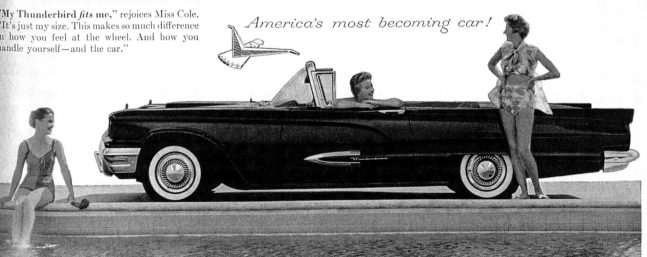

America's most becoming car!

How Anne Cole earned her T-bird.

In 1982, about ten years after Felligi retired, Anne Cole decided to try her own hand at designing. Rather than see her launch a rival label, Kayser-Roth worked out a deal whereby she could remain on staff and create the Cole Collection. She's still designing today, at an age she only describes as "somewhere between 50 and Forest Lawn." The collection is marketed by the latest corporate iteration, Authentic Fitness.

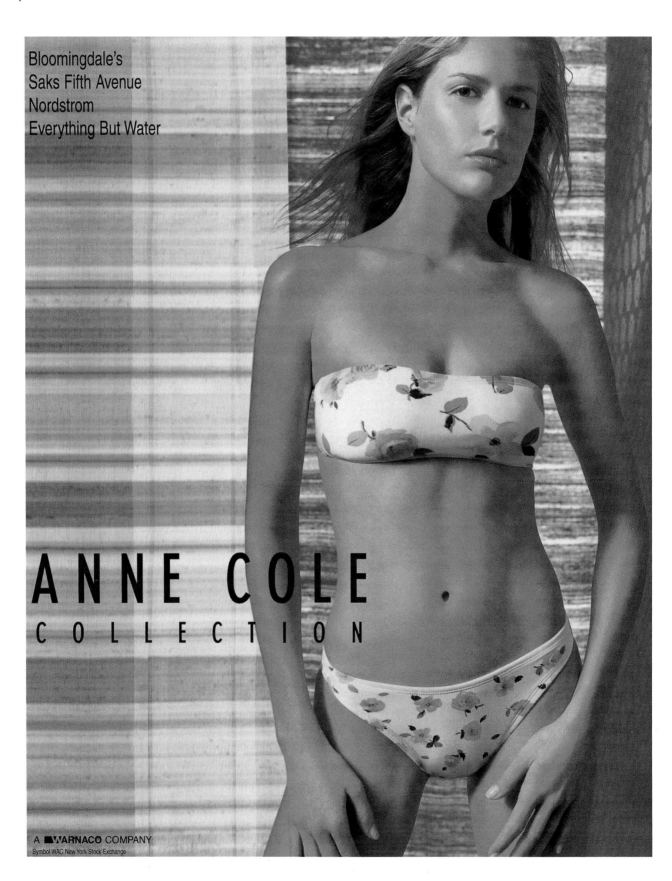

Bloomingdale's
Saks Fifth Avenue
Nordstrom
Everything But Water

ANNE COLE
COLLECTION

A ■WARNACO COMPANY
Symbol WAC New York Stock Exchange

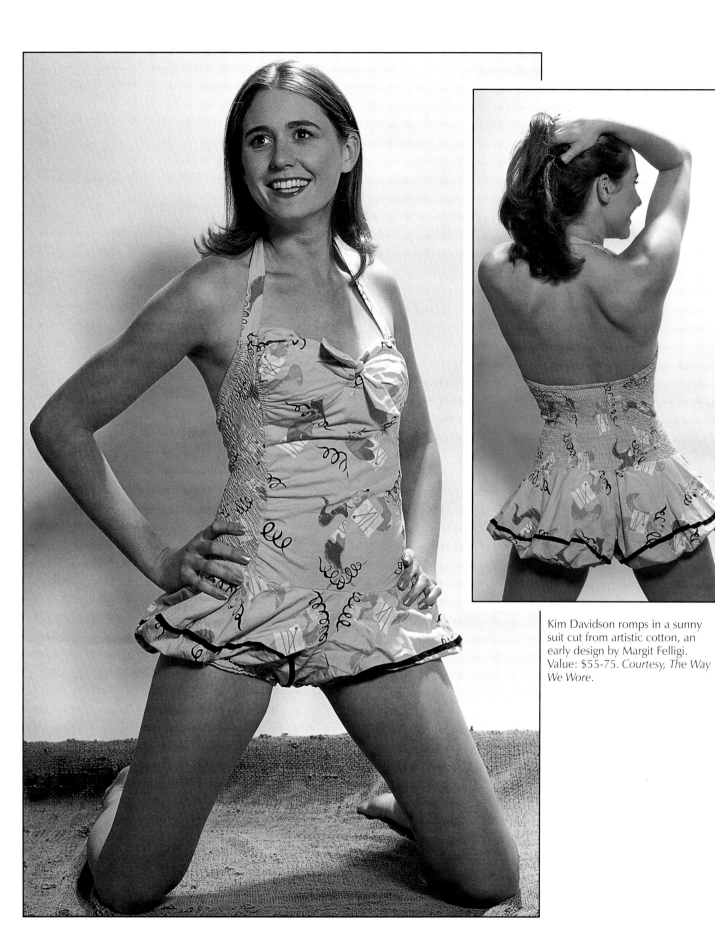

Kim Davidson romps in a sunny suit cut from artistic cotton, an early design by Margit Felligi. Value: $55-75. *Courtesy, The Way We Wore.*

Opposite page
Anne Cole touts the tankini as the first new swimwear silhouette to emerge in years. The bandeau bikini is another, shown here from her namesake collection for Summer 2000.

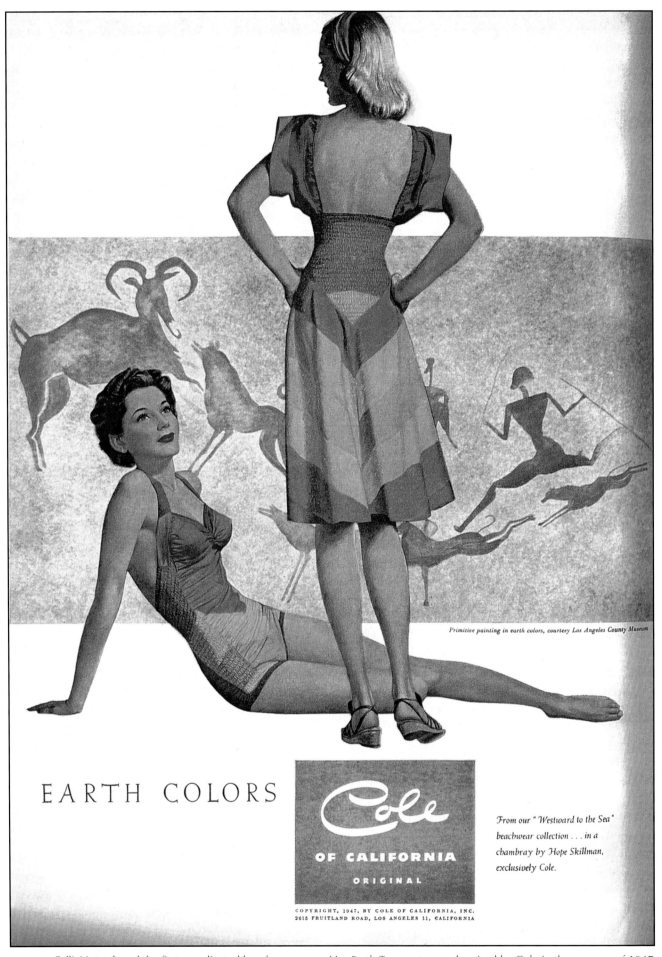

Felligi introduced the first coordinated beach cover-ups. Her *Earth Tones* set was advertised by Cole in the summer of 1947.

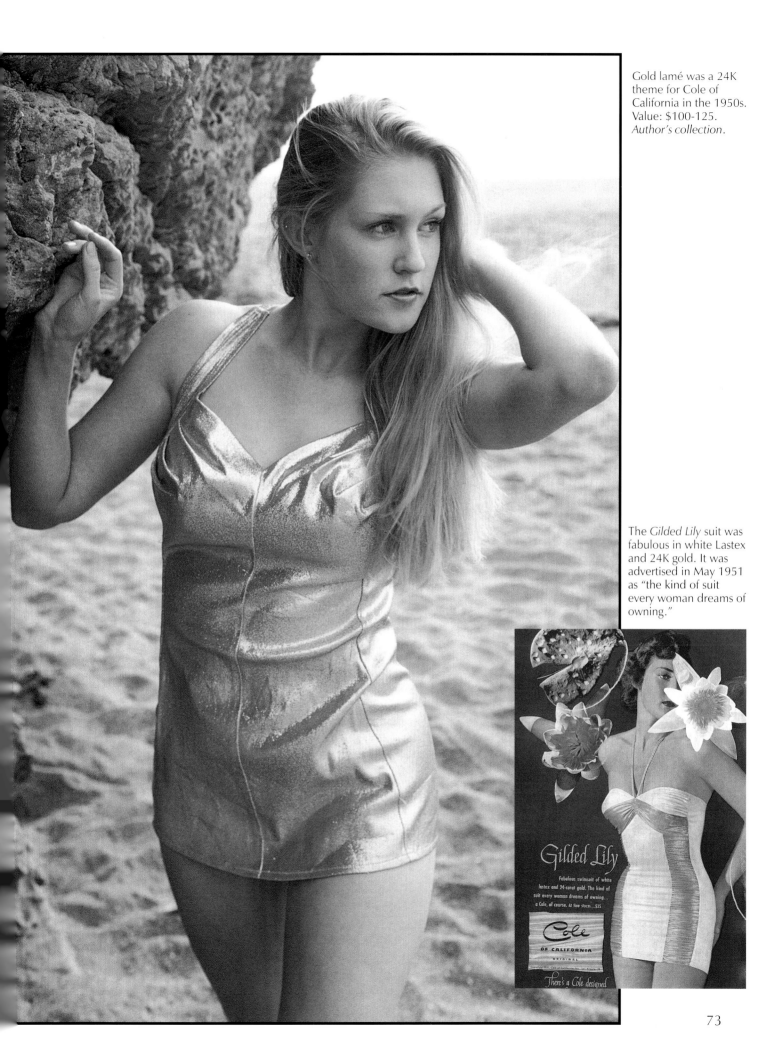

Gold lamé was a 24K theme for Cole of California in the 1950s. Value: $100-125. *Author's collection.*

The *Gilded Lily* suit was fabulous in white Lastex and 24K gold. It was advertised in May 1951 as "the kind of suit every woman dreams of owning."

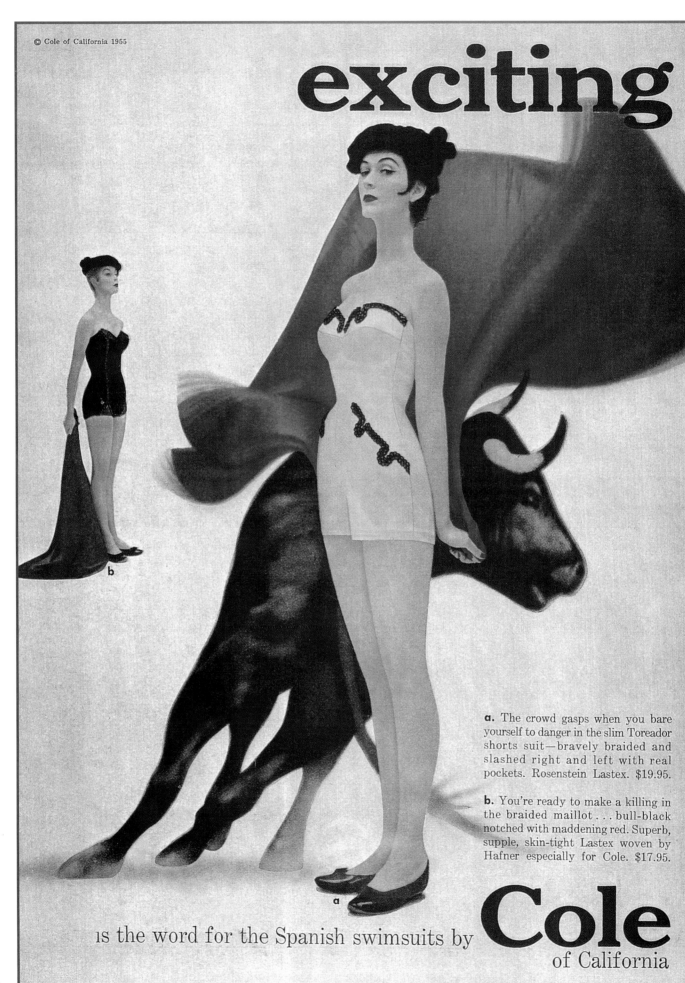

exciting

a. The crowd gasps when you bare yourself to danger in the slim Toreador shorts suit—bravely braided and slashed right and left with real pockets. Rosenstein Lastex. $19.95.

b. You're ready to make a killing in the braided maillot . . . bull-black notched with maddening red. Superb, supple, skin-tight Lastex woven by Hafner especially for Cole. $17.95.

is the word for the Spanish swimsuits by **Cole** of California

74

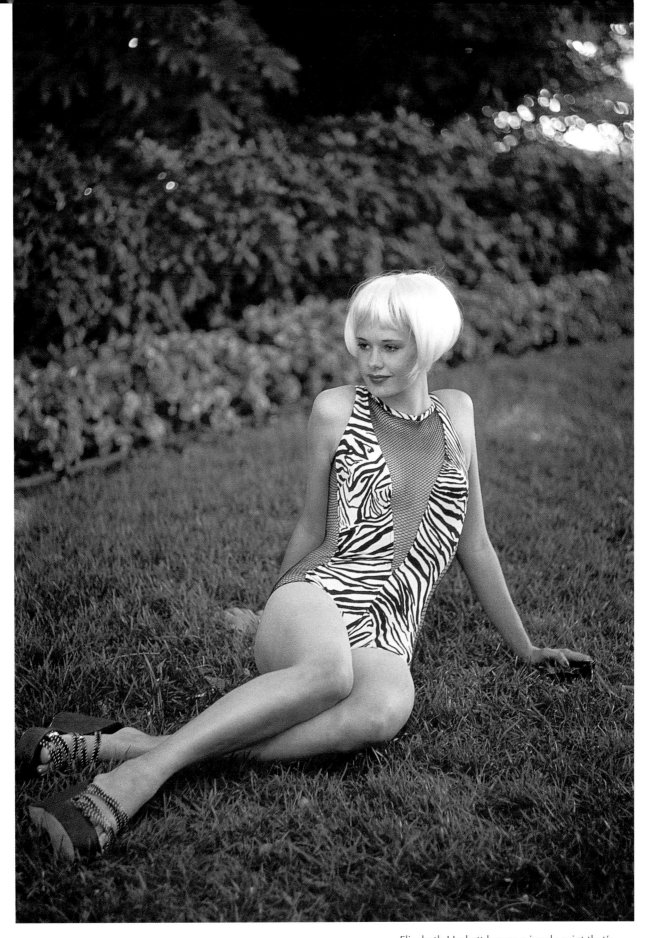

Elizabeth Haskett braves a jungle print that's barely tamed by netting (see following page for the same *Scandal Suit* with cream netting). Value: $75-95. *Courtesy, Cherry*.

Opposite page
The Spanish collection of 1955 was cut from a special-order Lastex. The yellow *Toreador*, with functional braided pockets, sold for $19.95. Its "bull black" companion sold for $17.95.

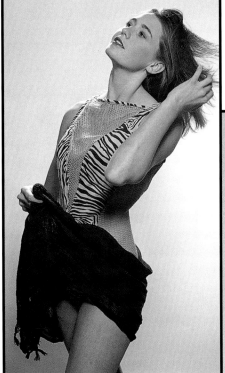

Kim Davidson creates another scandal: now you see it, now you don't. Value: $75-95. *Courtesy, The Way We Wore*.

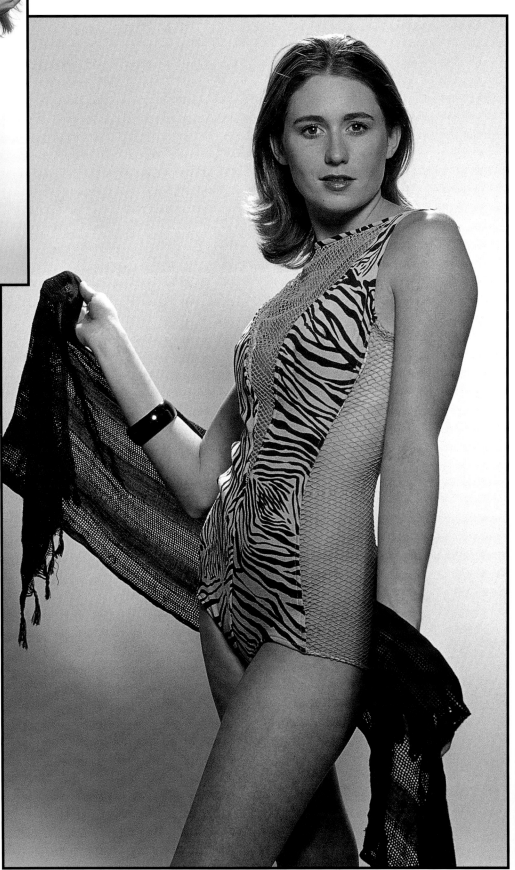

Opposite page
More wildcat styling in the Go Wild campaign of 1967.

76

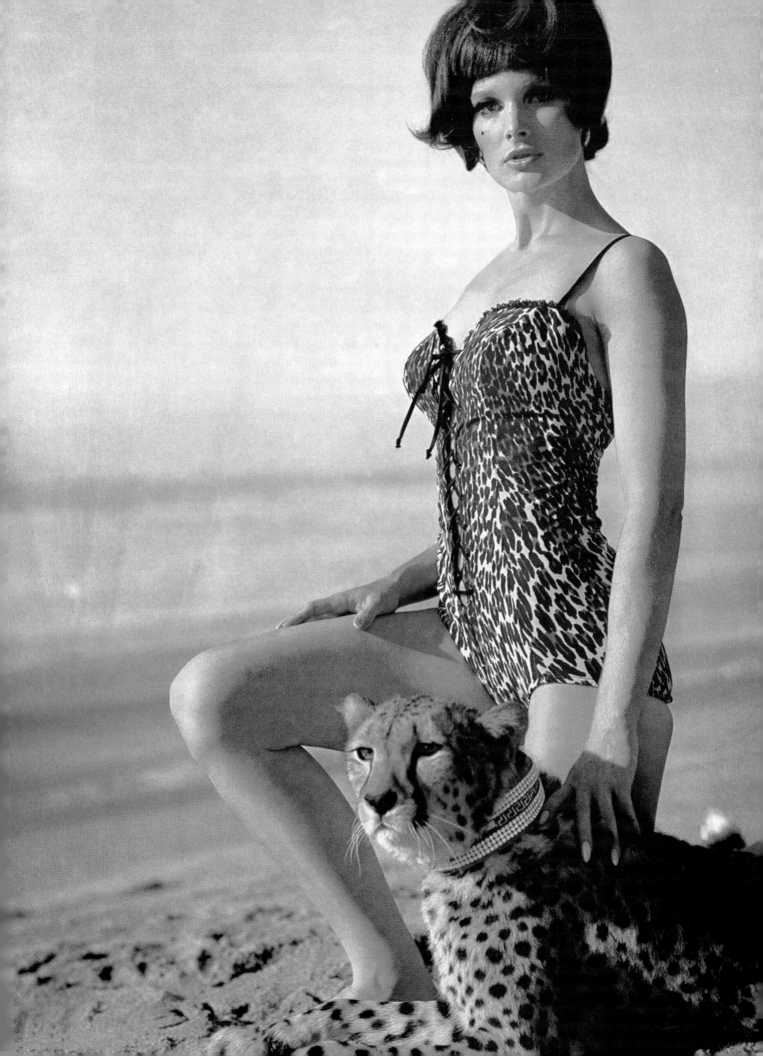

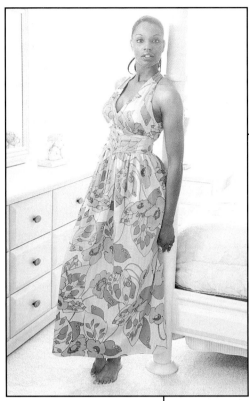

A white-hot floral print on a late 1970s jumpsuit, from one of Felligi's last collections. Value: $35-55. *Courtesy, Cheap Thrills.*

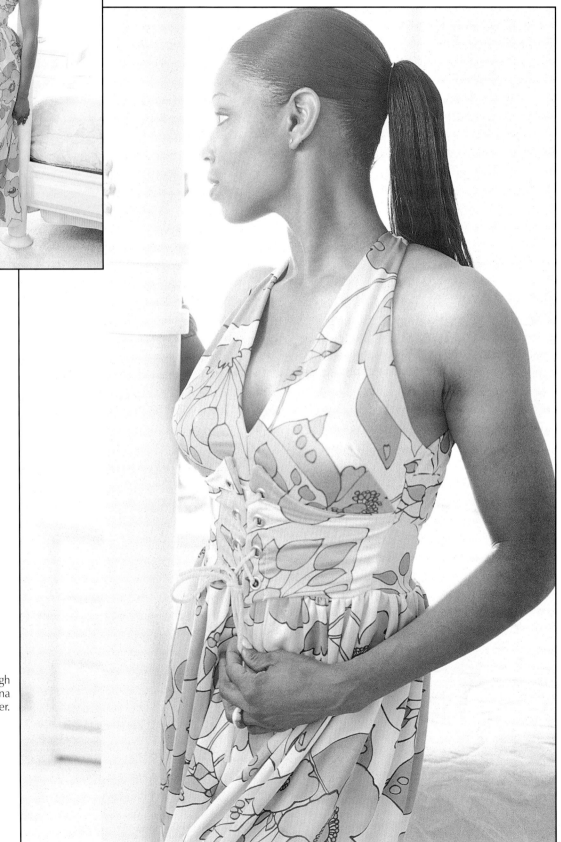

Corset detailing defines a high waistband on model Regina Alexander.

Catalina

By the 1930s, the industry was all about Jantzen, Catalina, and Cole. The three so dominated production they were referred to (with not a little regret by rival firms) as the "Ford, Chrysler and GM" of the industry.

Catalina was the first giant to stride across American beaches in 1912. That's when the Bentz Knitting Mills in Los Angeles added swimsuits to its inventory and changed its name to Pacific Knitting Mills. Under its founder, E.W. Stewart, the new company immediately unveiled two important new styles for men: the bold *Chicken Suit*, its brief lines emphasized by horizontal striping; and the *Speed Suit*, an early maillot with deeply slashed armholes and sloped trunks. The near-backless *Rib Stitch 5* followed for the distaff set. A sleekly functional silhouette, it would dominate American beaches for the remainder of the decade. Things were going swimmingly in 1928, when Stewart changed the name to Catalina.

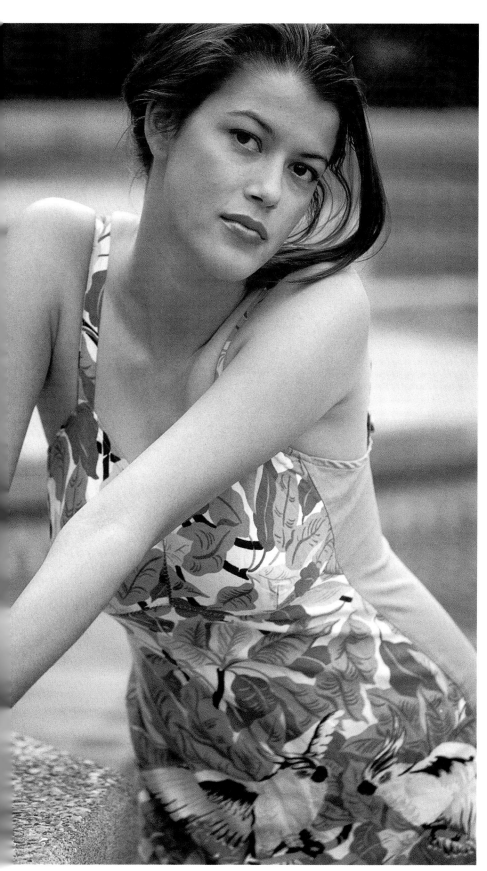

Chrystal Williams is all allure in this front panel suit. It's a Lastex fabric hand-blocked with jungle Cockatoos. Value: $95-125. *Courtesy, Luxe.*

Although Catalina shared many important attributes with the other West Coast giants, when it came to design there were clear distinctions. Jantzen was sporty and reliable, as befits a company founded on competition swimwear, and Cole was glamorous . But Catalina struck a middle ground, producing season-after-season of swimsuits designed to suit every taste—with a dash of spice.

Sometimes, however, the seasoning was left out. One of the company's most famous designs was a rather bland one-piece suit with a front panel. Originally designed for the Miss America Beauty Pageant in 1922, the panel was meant to be chaste, but it focused attention on the crotch! Nevertheless, it would be the reigning style of beauty queens for decades to come. Thanks to Stewart's skill in wangling the endorsement of pageant officials, Catalina was assured of a marketplace in the sun.

Even with its pageant honors, Catalina paid homage to Hollywood. In the late 1940s, Mary Ann DeWeese headed a "dream team" of costume designers: Milo Anderson and Orry Kelly from Warner Brothers, Edith Head from Paramount, and Howard Shoup from MGM, among others.

Catalina's "Hollywood Dream Team."

by TRAVIS BANTON
Universal International Studios

One of Seven World-Famous Hollywood Studio Designers* Creating for Catalina

* Catalina's 1947 Collecti
designed by Travis Banto
Universal Internation
Studios; Milo Anderso
Warner Brothers Picture
Inc.; Edith Head, Pa
mount Pictures, In
Howard Shoup, who b
designed for stars of Metr
Goldwyn-Mayer; Ve
West, Universal Inte
national Studios; Rem
RKO Radio Pictures, In
Edward Stevenson, RK
Radio Pictures, Inc. —
designing in collaborati
with Mary Ann DeWee
Catalina's Head Design

california in a swim suit

Color is California's special magic . . . subtle, bright, gay. They're all in your dramatic new Catalinas dramatized in exciting new designs by the unparalleled stylists of the cinema. Above: Travis Banton of Universal International Studios styles a one-piece suit in a classic mood in Mallinson's California Wild Flower print on rayon jersey. $10. Write for name of nearest store.

A Mallinson FABRIC

LOOK FOR T
FLYING FI

Catalina

TALINA SWIM SUITS • SWIM TRUNKS • SWEATERS
ina, Inc., Dept. 254, 443 So. San Pedro St., Los Angeles 13, California, U. S. A.

The company designer, Mary Ann DeWeese, began her career as a seamstress for Los Angeles Knitting Mills, where she learned the "knits and purls" of a technical trade. After turning her hand successfully to design she started the Sandeze label of sportswear. Somewhere along the line, she joined the swimwear division at Bentz Knitting Mills.

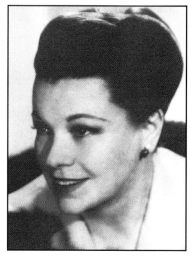

Mary Ann DeWeese.

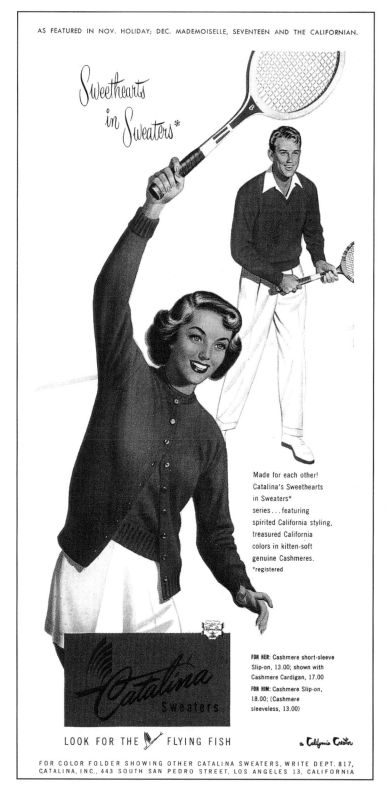

Catalina was always highly diversified. Even after its swimwear profile came into pageant prominence, the company continued to produce knit sportswear groups each season. Sporty sweaters for golf and tennis led to casual knit suits and knit separates until, in 1969, Catalina split into three separate divisions: swimwear, spectator sportswear, and active sportswear. By then, like Cole, it had been bought by Kayser-Roth. Each division was run as a separate company but they all retained a close liaison with the knitting mills.

Catalina included sweaters in its repertoire. This 1949 *Sweethearts in Sweaters* tennis duo shows a DeWeese innovation.

DeWeese is credited with innovations in the use of texture, including Jacquard knits and appliquéd stretch cottons. She also introduced "sweetheart" swimsuits and matching sportswear for men and women. Like Felligi at Cole, she designed pretty and practical beach cover-ups each season.

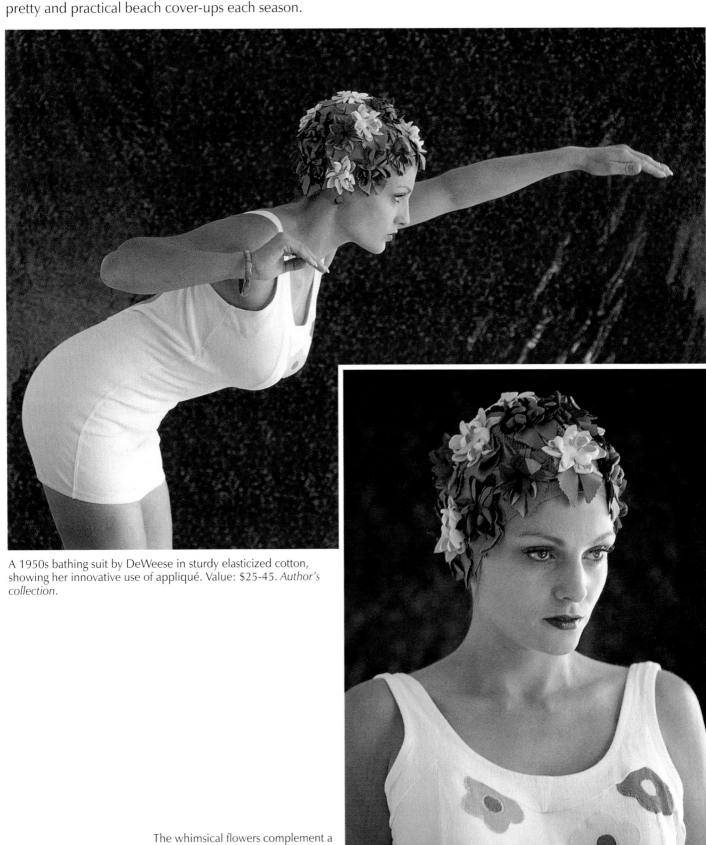

A 1950s bathing suit by DeWeese in sturdy elasticized cotton, showing her innovative use of appliqué. Value: $25-45. *Author's collection*.

The whimsical flowers complement a vintage swimcap.

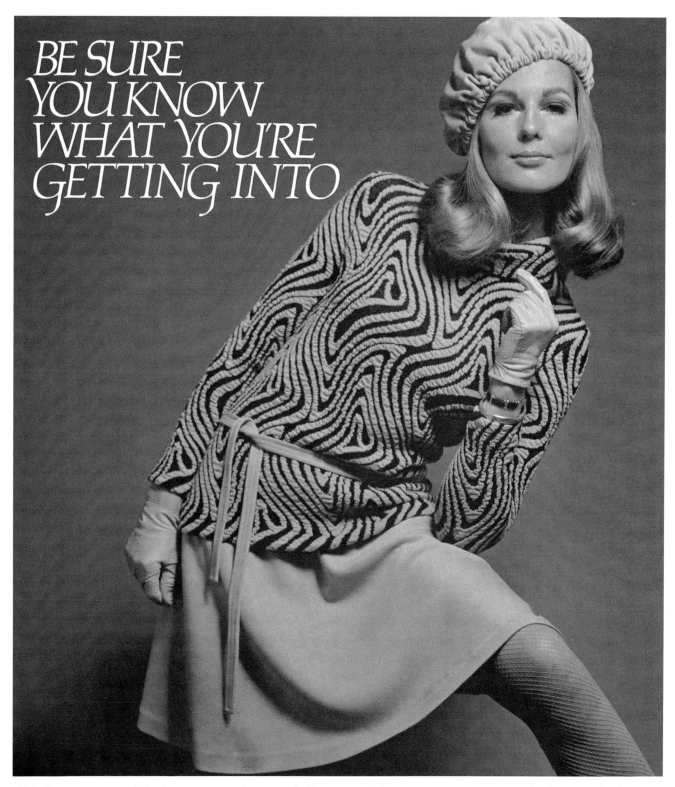

BE SURE
YOU KNOW
WHAT YOU'RE
GETTING INTO

With separates it's hang together or fall apart. When a customer comes in for a swinging skirt, that's that…unless she sees one of Catalina's color-related tops hanging right beside it. Then you can bet she'll buy both. So why get hung up hanging pants here and tops there? Hang together. Your customers will get the hang fast. And you'll be sure to get multiple sales.

BE SURE IT'S *Catalina*®

In later years, the company went mod. This swingin' three-piece set was advertised in 1970. Note the Mary Ann DeWeese legacy, a Jacquard top.

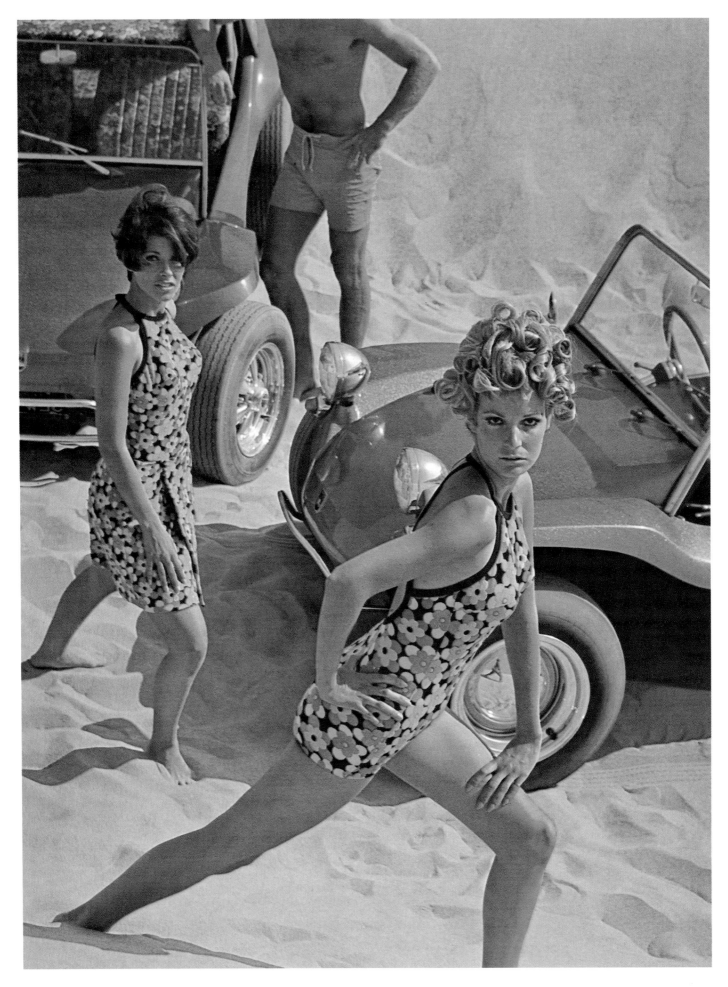

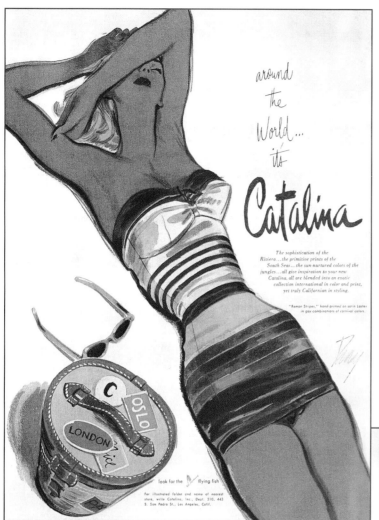

around the World... it's

Catalina

The sophistication of the Riviera...the primitive prints of the South Seas...the sun-nurtured colors of the jungles...all give inspiration to your new Catalina, all are blended into an exotic collection international in color and print, yet truly Californian in styling.

"Roman Stripes," hand-printed on satin Lastex in gay combinations of carnival colors.

look for the flying fish

For illustrated folder and name of nearest store, write Catalina, Inc., Dept. 310, 443 S. San Pedro St., Los Angeles, Calif.

Two strapless sunbathers, circa 1955. The ruffler is from a Caribbean Collection that featured fabrics by Jim Tillett of Mexico City. The striped *Riviera* is in hand-printed satin Lastex.

Opposite page
An appliquéd maillot and matching sundress by DeWeese, fun for surfing in 1967.

ventually founding her own business under the namesake label "DeWeese," she specialized in sundresses and loungers. In 1960, she designed diving suits for the U.S. Olympic team, a real tribute to her technical proficiency. Indeed, even the flirtiest DeWeese suit was clearly meant to *swim* in, and every dress or lounger featured the comfort of a built-in bra.

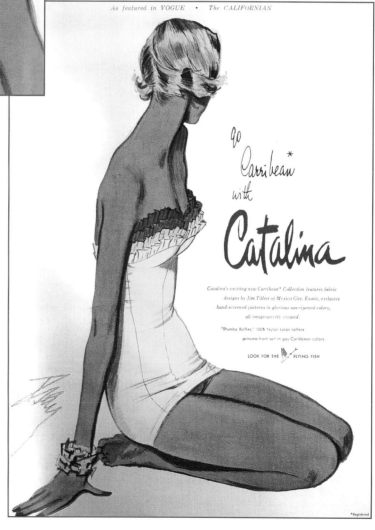

As featured in VOGUE • The CALIFORNIAN

go Carribean* with

Catalina

Catalina's exciting new Carribean Collection features fabric designs by Jim Tillett of Mexico City. Exotic, exclusive hand-screened patterns in glorious sun-ripened colors, all imaginatively created.*

"Rhumba Ruffles," 100% Nylon Lastex taffeta princess front suit in gay Caribbean colors.

LOOK FOR THE FLYING FISH

*Registered

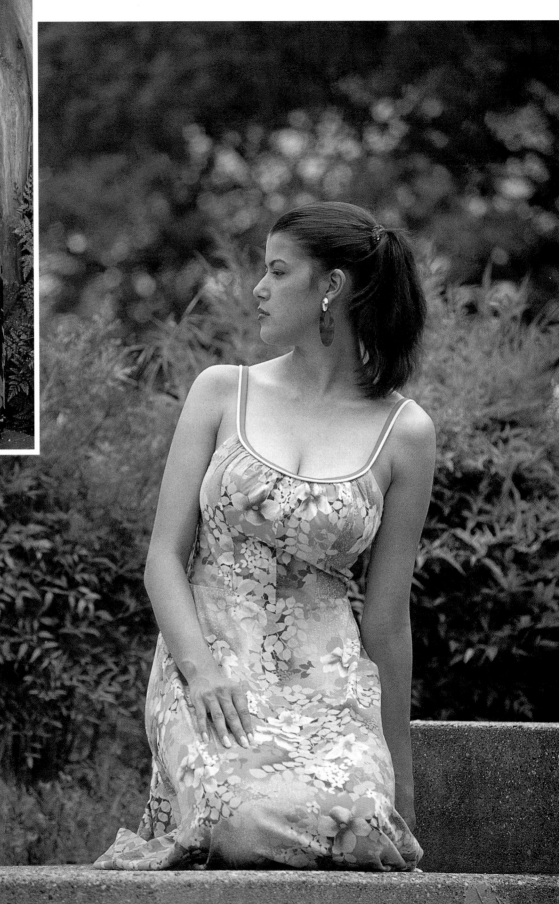

Fantasy flowers are a lush counterpoint to the simple lines of a rayon slip-dress, circa 1975 (scarf added). Value: $45-65. *Courtesy, Renaissance.*

This simple cotton sundress is made glamorous by décolletage. A built-in bra lends support. Value: $25-35. *Author's collection.*

After DeWeese struck off on her own, Catalina retained a series of designers, notably Bettina Jaynes, whose line was marked by an ethnic sensibility in keeping with the hip fashions of the day. She worked for Catalina in the late 1960s under Karl Kluth. When he left to found the Marilyn K. line of casual wear in the spring of 1969, she followed him as head designer for the new company.

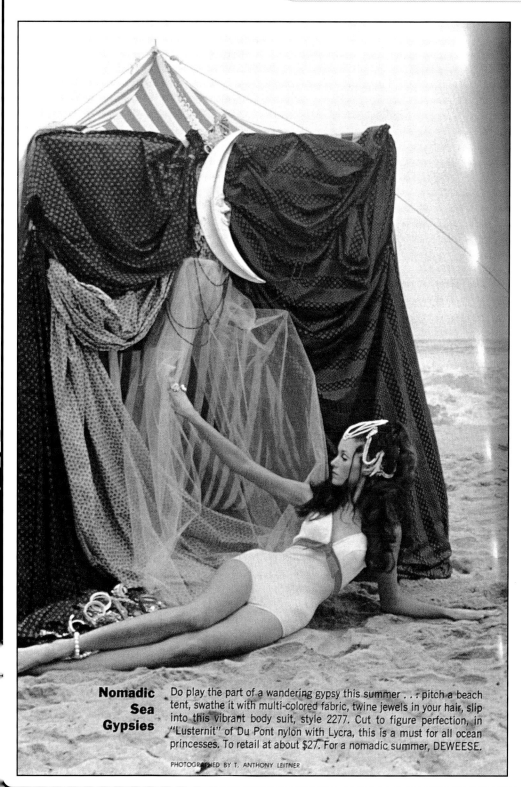

Nomadic Sea Gypsies Do play the part of a wandering gypsy this summer . . . pitch a beach tent, swathe it with multi-colored fabric, twine jewels in your hair, slip into this vibrant body suit, style 2277. Cut to figure perfection, in "Lusternit" of Du Pont nylon with Lycra, this is a must for all ocean princesses. To retail at about $27. For a nomadic summer, DEWEESE.

PHOTOGRAPHED BY T. ANTHONY LEITNER

In Fall 1968, this ad exhorted readers to "play the part of a wandering gypsy this summer" in a parti-color suit by Bettina Jaynes.

It's no wonder that Elisabeth (Bette) Stewart, having been raised in the business as the daughter of Catalina's founder, gravitated to a career in sportswear design. In 1955, with her husband Robert Beck and her two brothers David and Bill, she founded Elisabeth Stewart Swimwear in Los Angeles.

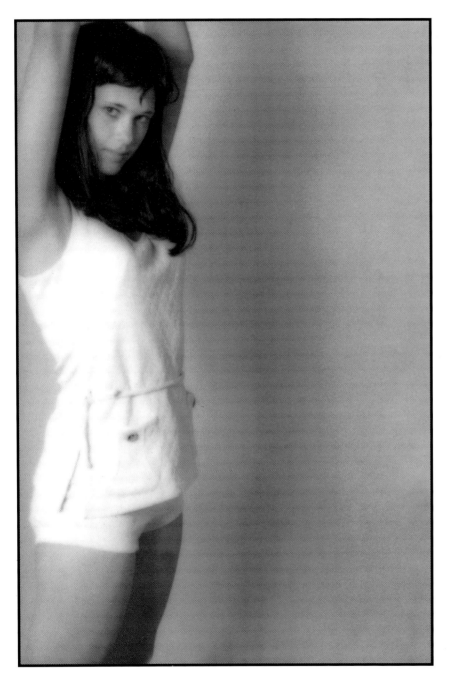

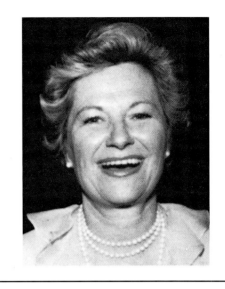

Elisabeth Stewart

Elisabeth Stewart, designing daughter.

Pick a daffodil yellow shell top and boy shorts, a perky duo from the mid-1960s. Value: $45-55. *Author's collection*.

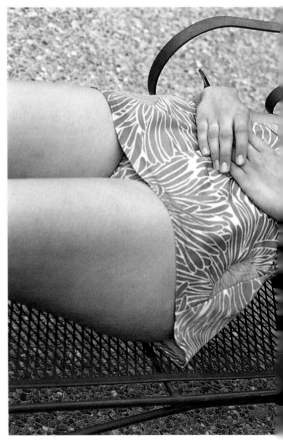

Stewart's eminently wearable suits, with motifs borrowed from Mary Ann DeWeese's design lexicon, were popular throughout the 1960s. She was recognized for her design achievement with the coveted Coty American Fashion Critic's Award for sportswear.

Tall-stemmed pink roses bloom on Kim Davidson.
This white cotton swimsuit is cut like a jumper. By
Elisabeth Stewart, circa 1965. Value: $35-45.
Courtesy, Luxe.

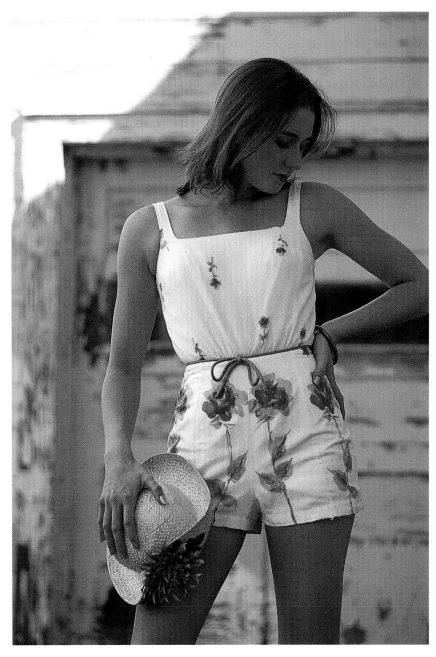

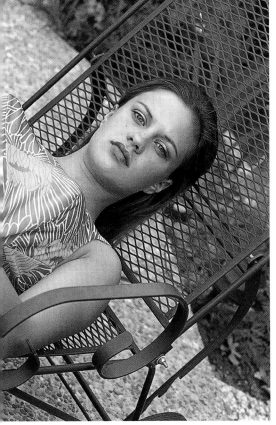

An elasticized maillot by Elisabeth Stewart, with
Catalina's signature panel skirt. Value: $35-45.
Courtesy, Luxe.

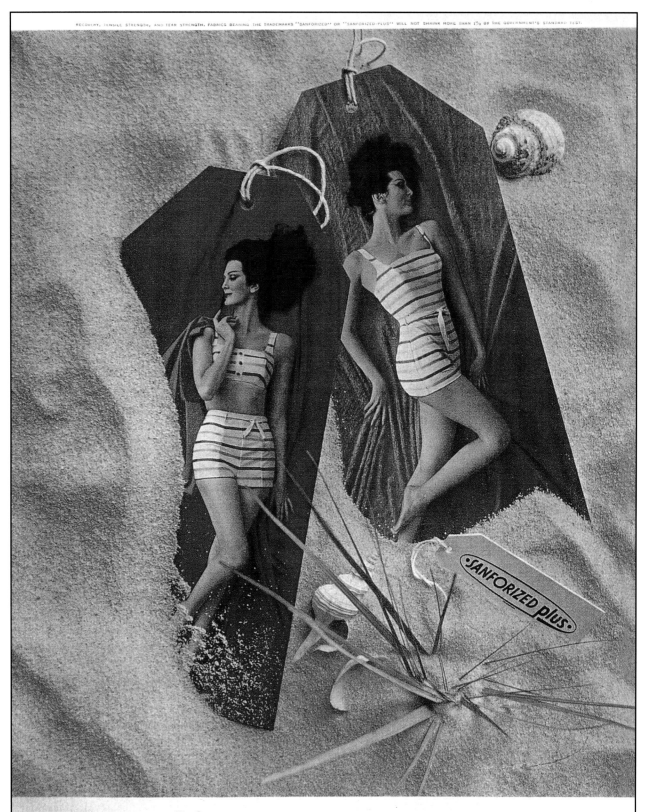

Relax... you'll never be in better shape for summer

ELISABETH STEWART keeps you stunning while sunning... in swim suits tailored of satin-striped woven-check cotton. Fashion conscious suits that hold their shape (and make yours look even better). Protected against wrinkles, creases, shrinkage by the **SANFORIZED-PLUS** label. ■ Nectarine stripe on yellow, lime peel on blue. One-piece suit, sizes 10-18, about $20. Two-piece suit, sizes 8-16, about $19. At Bloomingdale's, New York; Carson, Pirie Scott, Chicago; D. H. Holmes, New Orleans; Joseph Magnin, San Francisco; Neiman-Marcus, Dallas; and J. W. Robinson's, Los Angeles.

Striped cotton suits were the ticket to fun for Resort 1962.

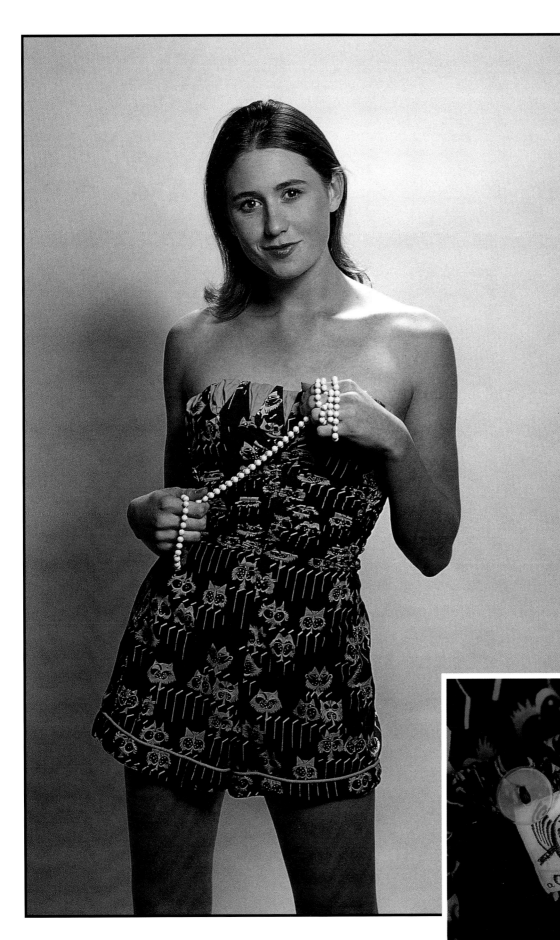

Pink pussycats peek-at-you from a black cotton romper suit, part of Catalina's earliest junior line. The fabric is attributed to Elza of Hollywood. Value: $75–95. *Courtesy, The Way We Wore.*

The first Catalina label had a capital "C" palette, and a flying fish paintbrush.

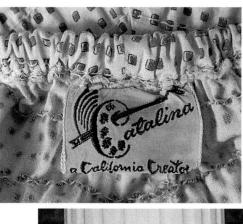

Styled for the Stars, circa 1955.

Orange stars and squares are perky on a white
bloomer suit. Value: $55-75. *Courtesy, The Way
We Wore.*

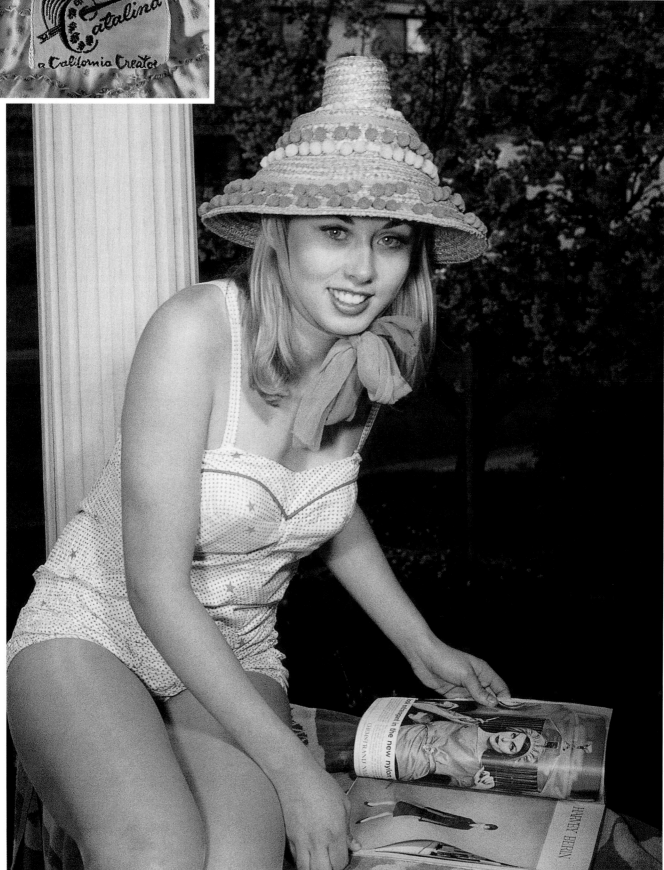

92

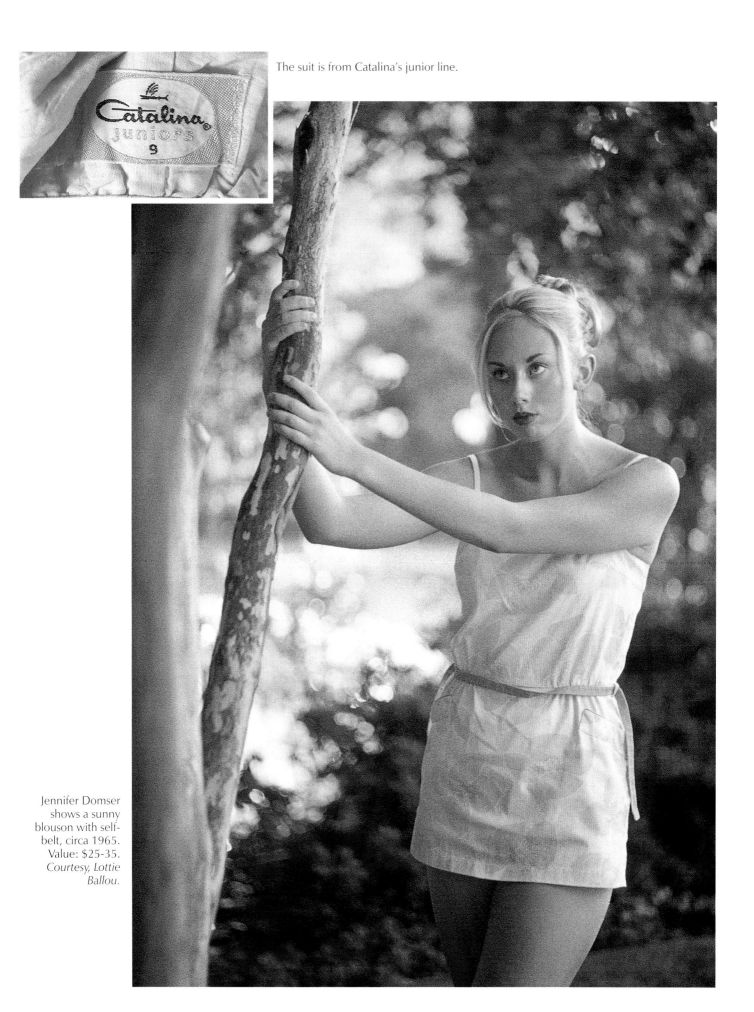

The suit is from Catalina's junior line.

Jennifer Domser
shows a sunny
blouson with self-
belt, circa 1965.
Value: $25-35.
*Courtesy, Lottie
Ballou.*

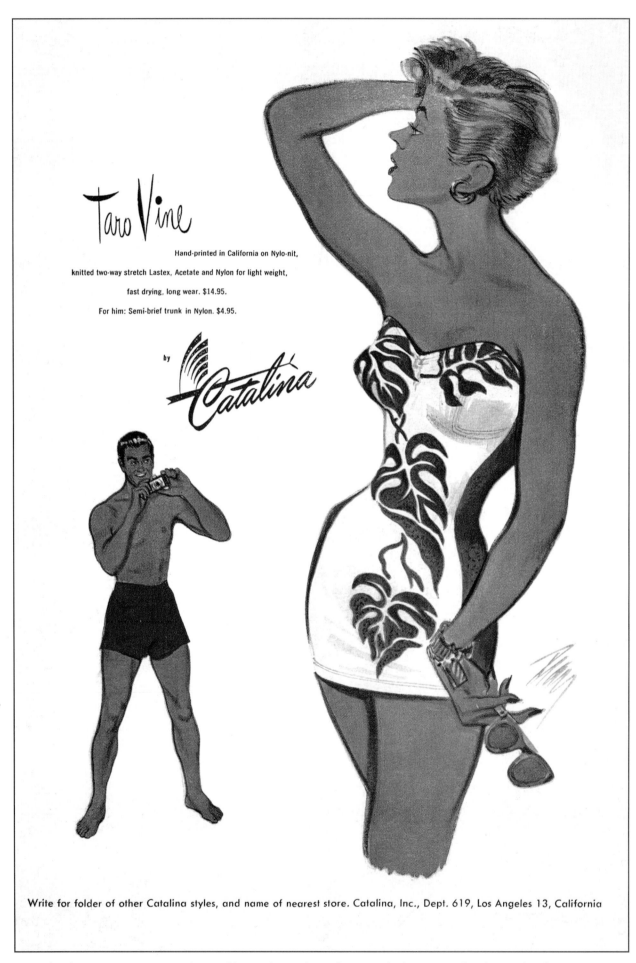

Taro Vine

Hand-printed in California on Nylo-nit,
knitted two-way stretch Lastex, Acetate and Nylon for light weight,
fast drying, long wear. $14.95.

For him: Semi-brief trunk in Nylon. $4.95.

by

Catalina

The divine *Taro Vine* suit, as advertised by Catalina in the mid-1950s. The leaves were hand printed on knit Lastex.

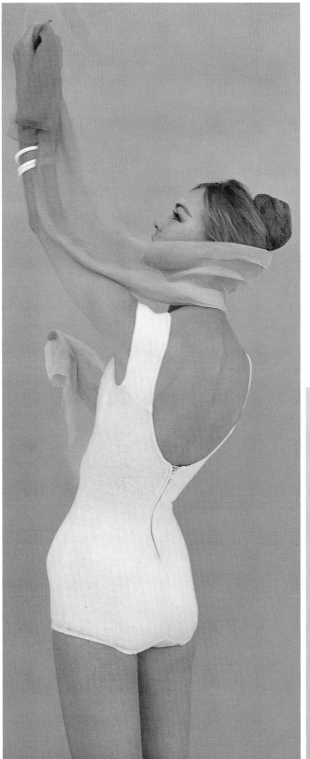

Such a simple maillot, in pure white knit.
It's a timeless style, but the metal zipper
dates this suit to the early 1960s.
Courtesy, Jimmy Mitchell.

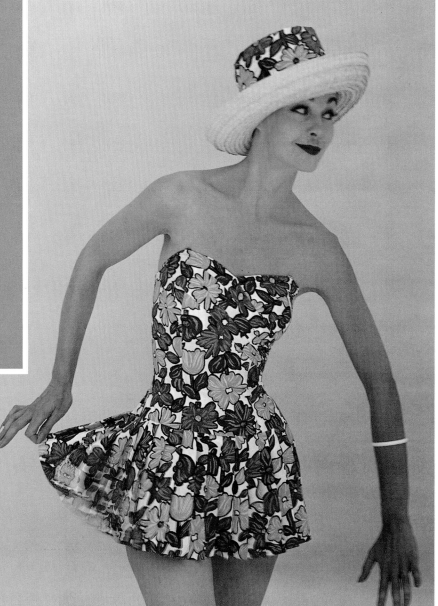

Sarong styling gives this sunny one-piece a tropical
tone. The styling is 1940s, but this is actually a late
1950s style. *Courtesy, Jimmy Mitchell.*

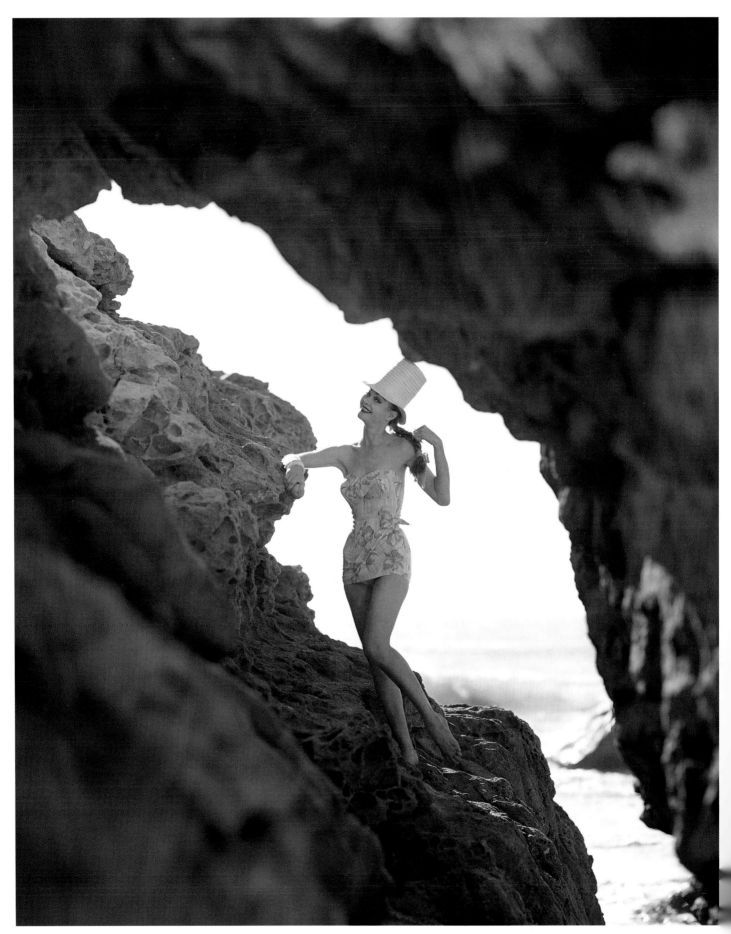

Everything's coming up sunshine in a skirted suit with
matching sunhat, circa 1960. *Courtesy, Jimmy Mitchell.*

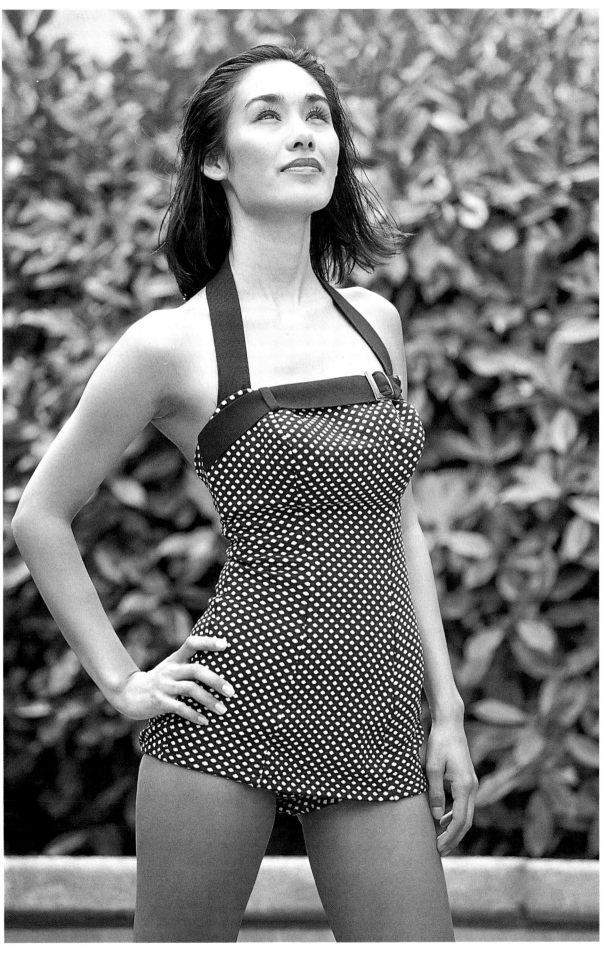

Kristi Talbert soaks in the sun in a one-piece knit suit, with a broad band of elastic as halter neckline (the buckle detail is typical of mid-1960s). Value: $25-35. *Author's collection.*

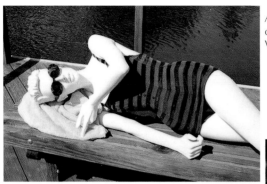

A top performer in black and taupe elasticized cotton. This suit was meant for sports, circa 1950. Value: $55-75. *Courtesy, The Way We Wore.*

Elizabeth Haskett wears a boy-cut suit by Catalina in a simple cotton print, from the mid-1950s. Value: $25-35. *Courtesy, Lottie Ballou.*

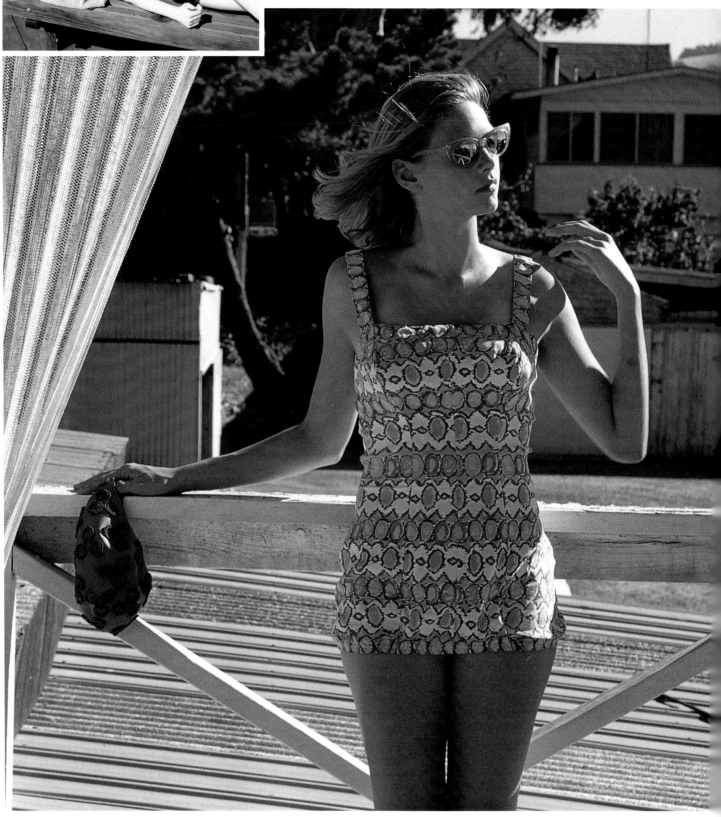

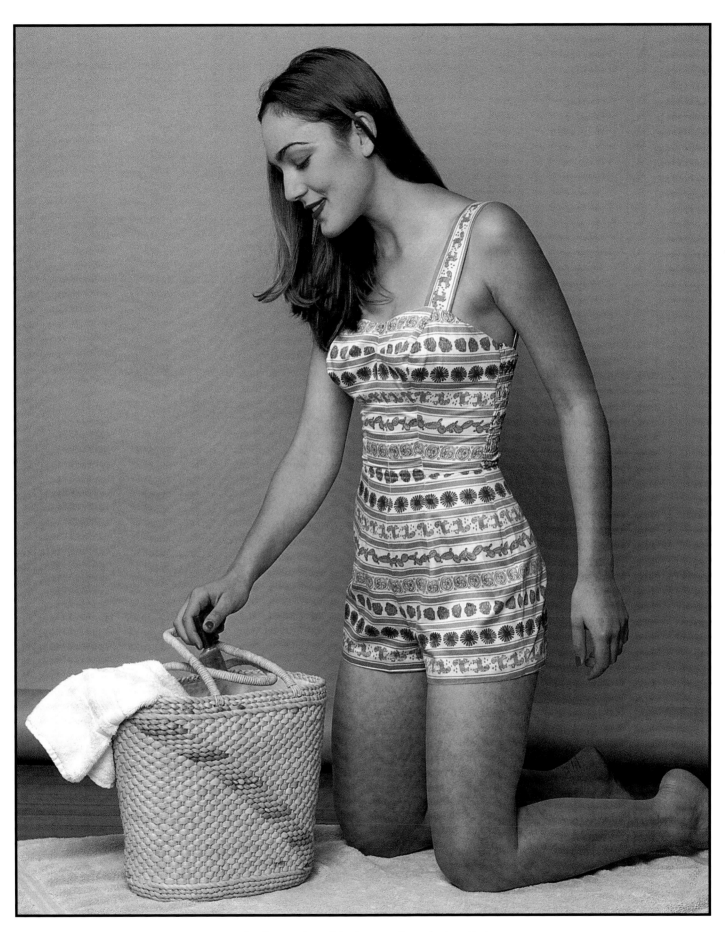

Another boy-cut in polished cotton, from the late 1950s, on
Monica Moreno. Value: $25-45. *Courtesy, Lottie Ballou.*

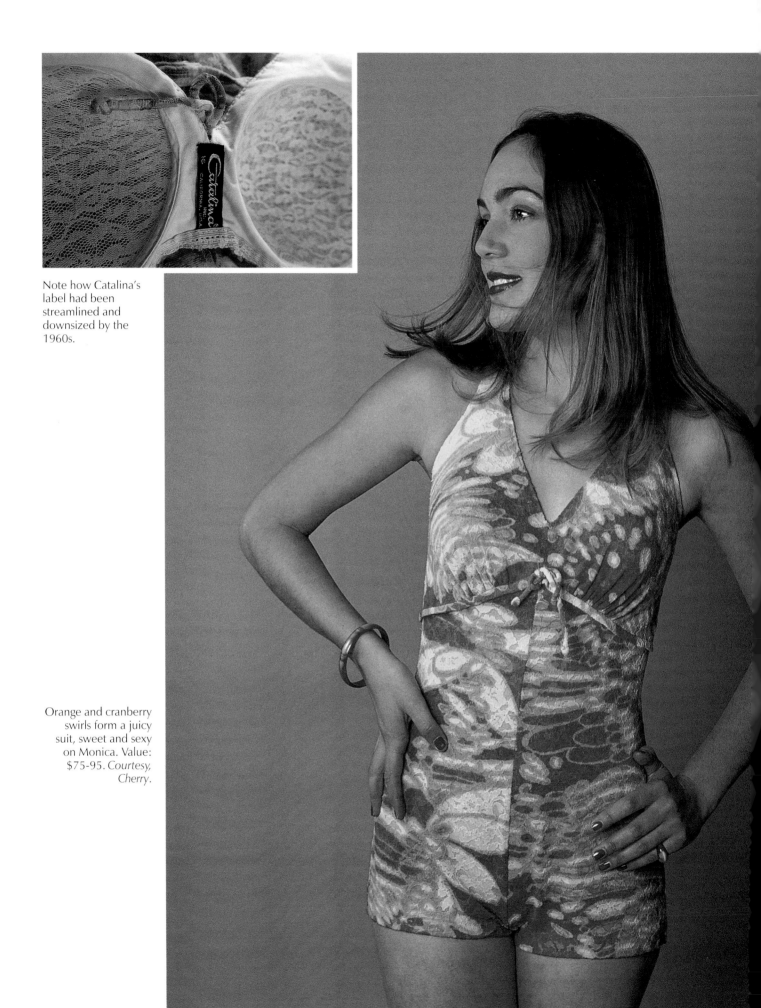

Note how Catalina's label had been streamlined and downsized by the 1960s.

Orange and cranberry swirls form a juicy suit, sweet and sexy on Monica. Value: $75-95. *Courtesy, Cherry*.

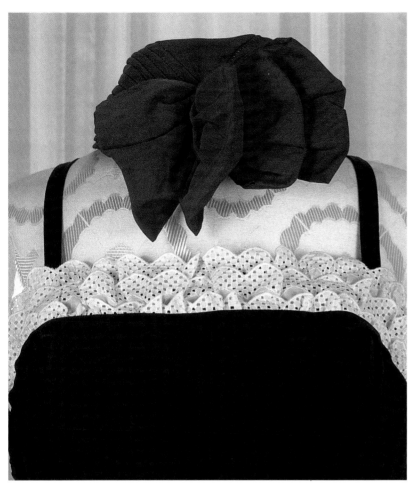

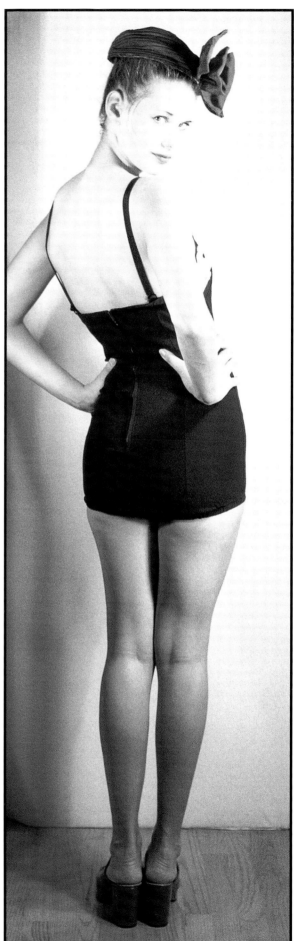

Elizabeth Haskett strikes a Betty Grable pose in this alluring Lastex swimsuit from Catalina, circa 1945. White eyelet trim was featured on the otherwise plain suit, shown here sparked by a raspberry bow-tie turban, same era. Value: $55-75. *Courtesy, The Way We Wore.*

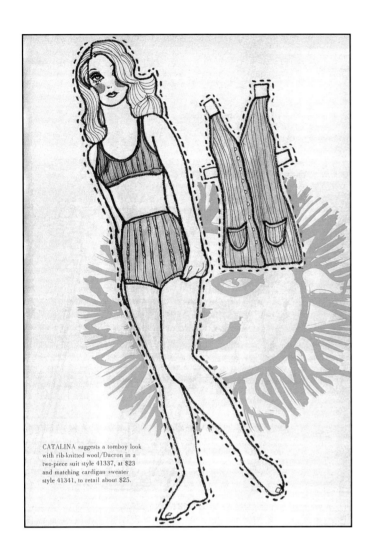

CATALINA suggests a tomboy look
with rib-knitted wool/Dacron in a
two-piece suit style 41337, at $23
and matching cardigan sweater
style 41341, to retail about $25.

Paper dolls are ready for play in a two-piecer by
Catalina and beach pants by DeWeese.

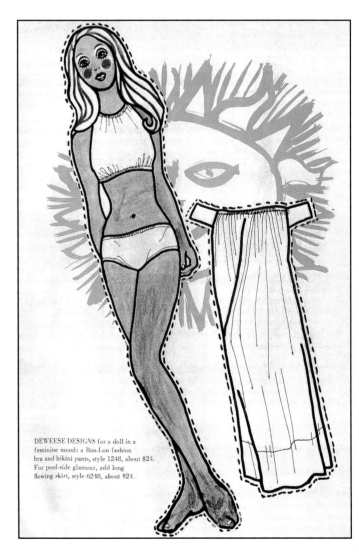

DEWEESE DESIGNS for a doll in a
feminine mood: a Ban-Lon fashion
bra and bikini pants, style 1248, about $24.
For pool-side glamour, add long
flowing skirt, style 6248, about $24.

Rose Marie Reid

Although Rose Marie Reid does not rank among the early giants, the swimwear industry was greatly influenced by the insouciant style

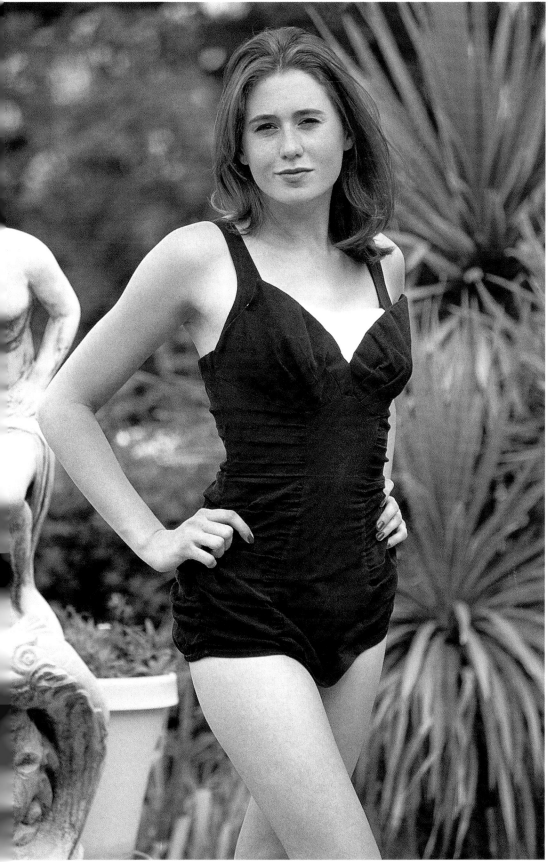

of this designer. Reid, a passionate swimmer from Vancouver, British Columbia, was so dissatisfied with the prevailing styles that she turned her seamstress talents to work and began a one-woman operation in 1937.

In her first year of business, Reid grossed $10,000, with most of her sales in western Canada. She released her first line to rave reviews at the pre-resort market week in Los Angeles, where buyers from the largest department stores were gathered to stock their racks of bathing suits. From that first season forward, the Rose Marie Reid label would set a new standard in swimwear.

An early Rose Marie Reid, all discreet flattery in shirred black Lastex. The peaked bra shows off a creamy modesty panel. Value: $35-55. *Courtesy, Luxe.*

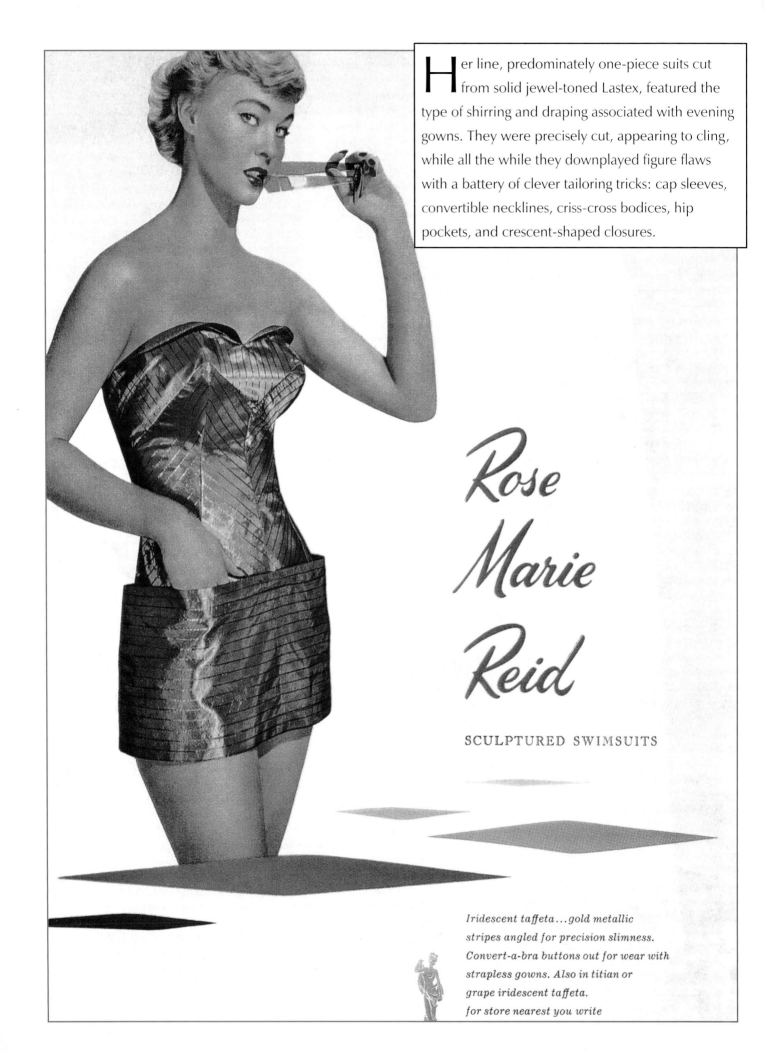

H er line, predominately one-piece suits cut from solid jewel-toned Lastex, featured the type of shirring and draping associated with evening gowns. They were precisely cut, appearing to cling, while all the while they downplayed figure flaws with a battery of clever tailoring tricks: cap sleeves, convertible necklines, criss-cross bodices, hip pockets, and crescent-shaped closures.

Rose Marie Reid

SCULPTURED SWIMSUITS

Iridescent taffeta...gold metallic stripes angled for precision slimness. Convert-a-bra buttons out for wear with strapless gowns. Also in titian or grape iridescent taffeta. for store nearest you write

Reid infused increasingly low-cut swim silhouettes with a sense of high class. It was still Hollywood glamour—but now it was in the manner of Grace Kelly, rather than Bridgit Bardot. Her style meshed perfectly with the postwar "return to normalcy" impetus that drove other ladylike trends in fashion. Soon, a Los Angeles couple seeking to back a new enterprise, Jack and Nina Kessler, contacted Reid with a proposal. By 1946, Kessler had financed the venture with $50,000 of his own money and established a distribution network throughout the United States. Reid's collateral was her talent, patents, and manufacturing expertise.

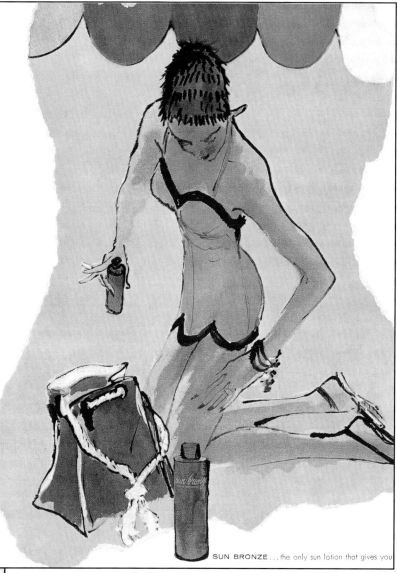

SUN BRONZE . . . the only sun lotion that gives you

Above: The *Moulin Rouge* suit, part of Rose Marie Reid's Couturier Collection in 1955—as sketched for a suntan lotion ad.

Left: The collection also featured *Spellbound* (at left, with gold studs) and *Roulette* (shown at right in amethyst; sapphire, magenta, and agate were other options).

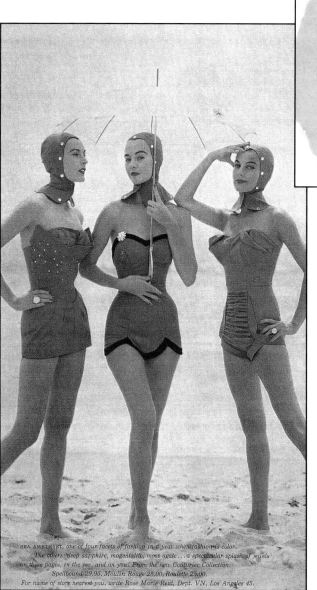

SEA AMETHYST, one of four facets of fashion in a year when fashion is color. The others: deep sapphire, magentalite, moss agate . . . a spectacular splash of jewels on these pages, in the sea, and on you! From the new Couturier Collection: Spellbound 29.95, Moulin Rouge 25.00, Roulette 25.00. For name of store nearest you, write Rose Marie Reid, Dept. VN, Los Angeles 45.

The New Look, Christian Dior's elegant styling that debuted as a collection in 1947, demanded a return to corseting, which was no problem for Rose Marie Reid suits with their built-in boning and girdle-like paneling. Although the New Look rapidly changed into a variety of new shapes for streetwear, Reid's look remained in favor for swimwear throughout the 1950s.

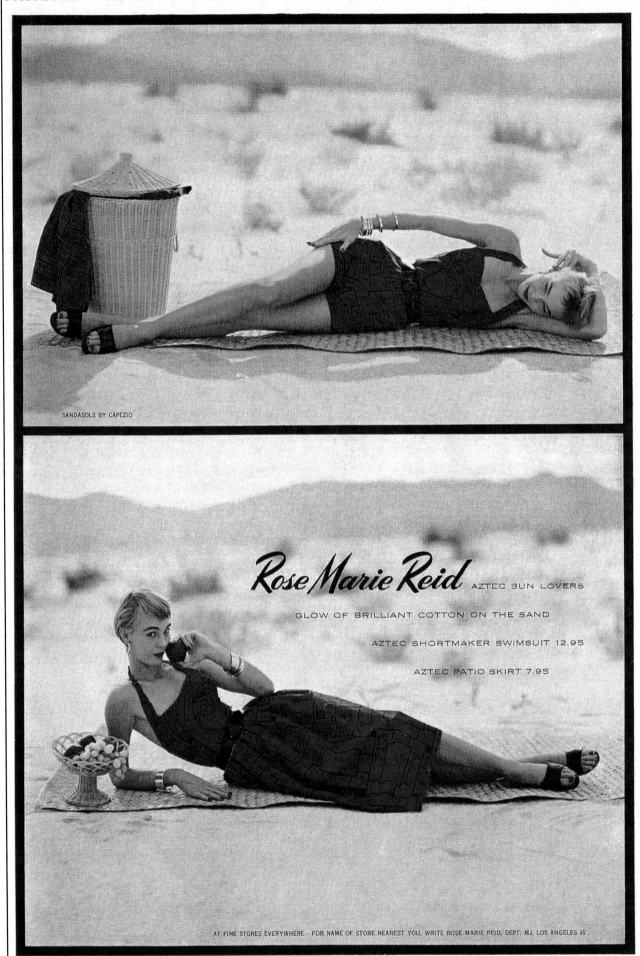

SANDASOLS BY CAPEZIO

Rose Marie Reid AZTEC SUN LOVERS

GLOW OF BRILLIANT COTTON ON THE SAND

AZTEC SHORTMAKER SWIMSUIT 12.95

AZTEC PATIO SKIRT 7.95

AT FINE STORES EVERYWHERE · FOR NAME OF STORE NEAREST YOU, WRITE ROSE MARIE REID, DEPT. MJ, LOS ANGELES 45

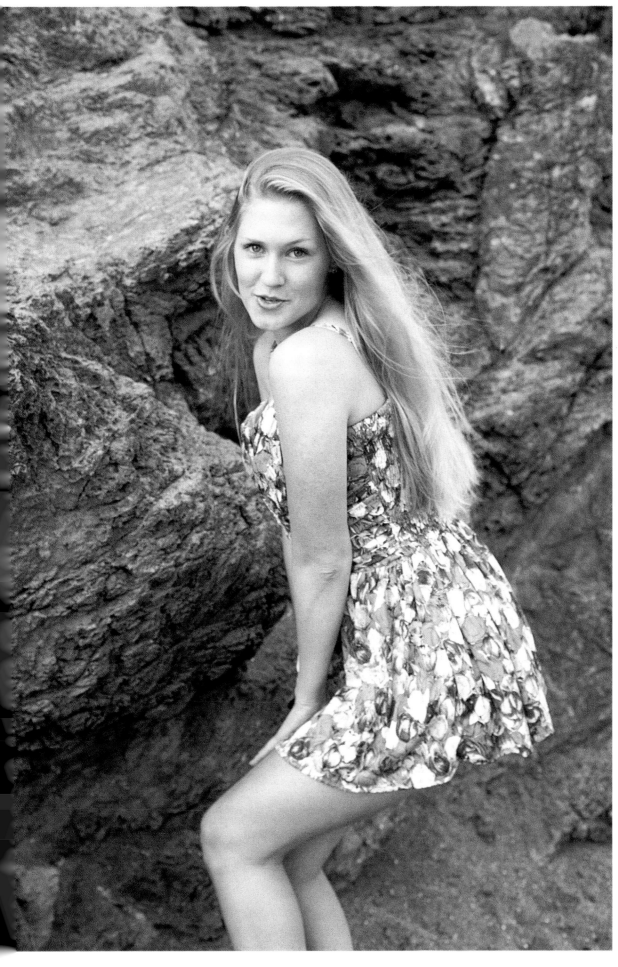

As much sundress as swimsuit, this rayon charmer took you from beach to barbeque in the mid-1950s. Value: $25-35. *Author's collection.*

Opposite page: The *Aztec Shortmaker* was $12.95; its companion *Aztec Patio Skirt* was $7.95, as marketed in the early 1950s.

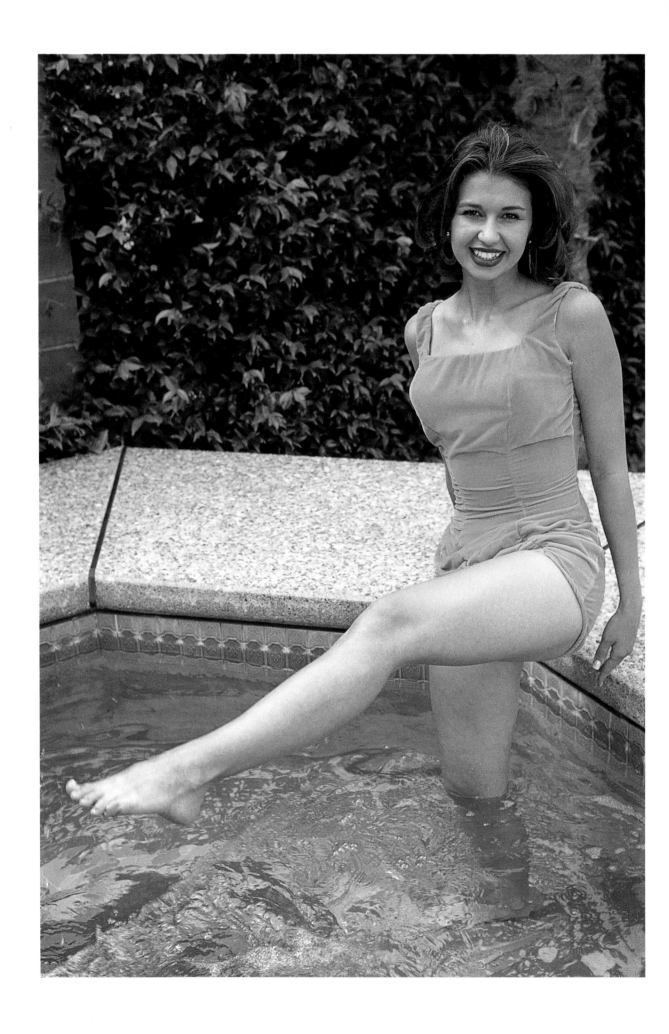

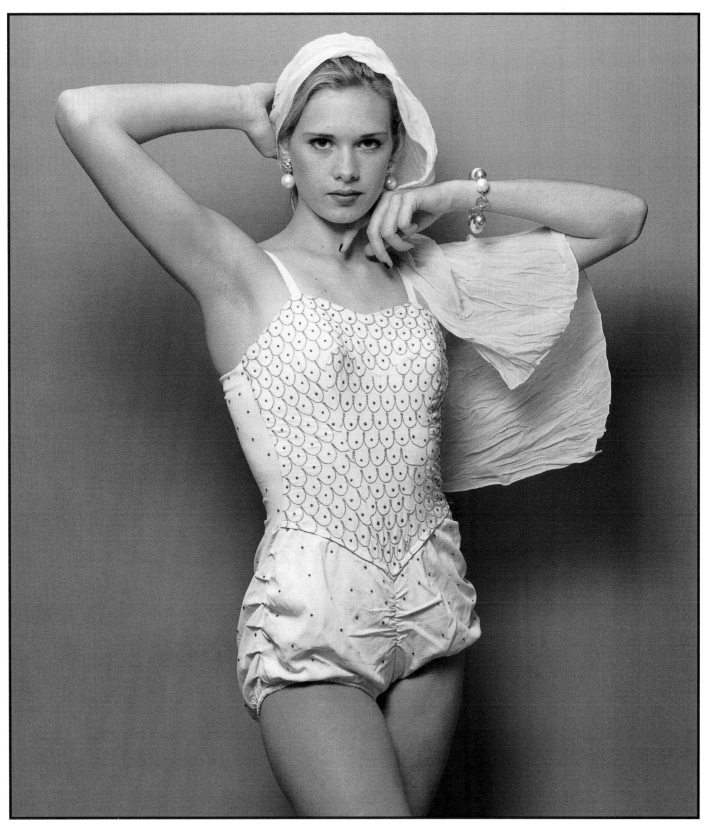

Gold soutache flirts on the bodice, studs wink from the bloomer bottom. All in all,
Elizabeth Haskett has all-out glamour in this mid-1950s suit by Rose Marie Reid.
Value: $65-75. *Courtesy, The Way We Wore.*

Opposite page
Tangerine was a hot color in the mid-1950s, shown
here in cotton velvet for Reid's Limited Edition label.
Value: $45-55. *Author's collection.*

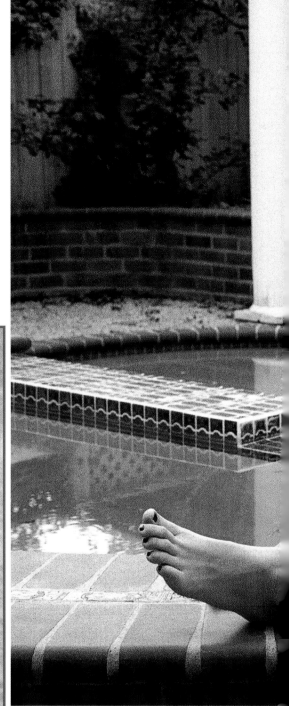

More glamour in a diamond-pattern Jacquard,
elasticized for fit and comfort. Value: $65-75.
Courtesy, The Way We Wore.

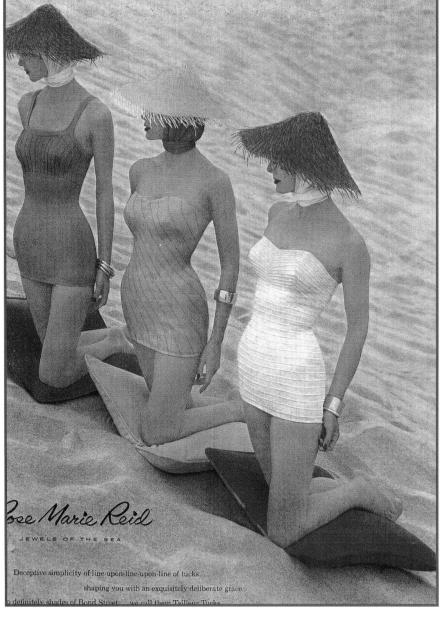

Rose Marie Reid

JEWELS OF THE SEA

Deceptive simplicity of line-upon-line-upon-line of tucks...

shaping you with an exquisitely deliberate grace.

...definitely shades of Bond Street... we call them Tailleur Tucks.

A line-up of fitted swimsuits by Rose
Marie Reid, dubbed *Tailleur Tucks*.
Gotta love those coolie sunhats!

110

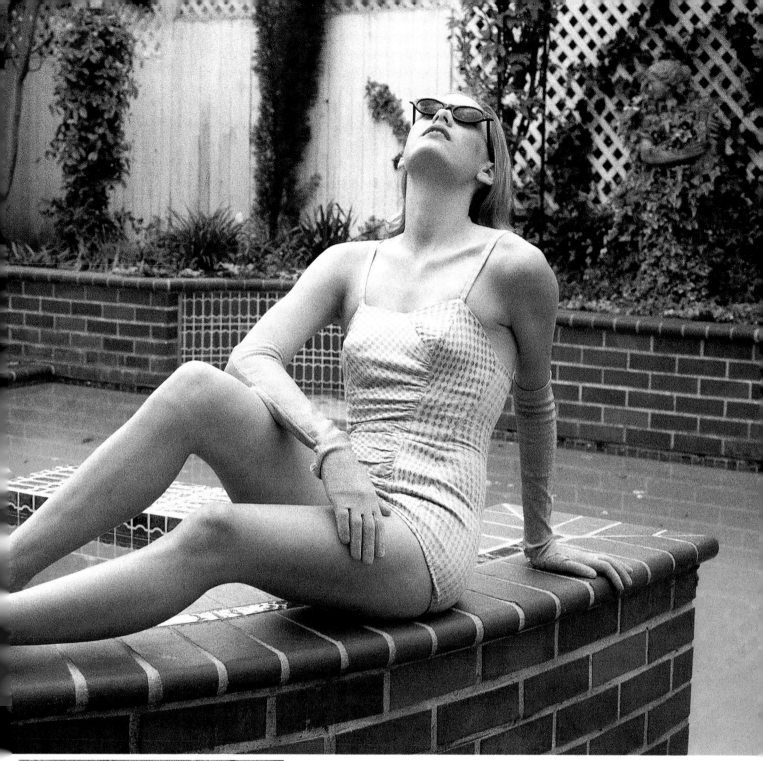

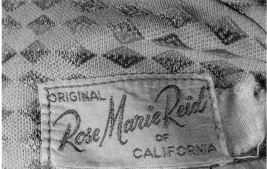

The Rose Marie Reid label, circa 1955.

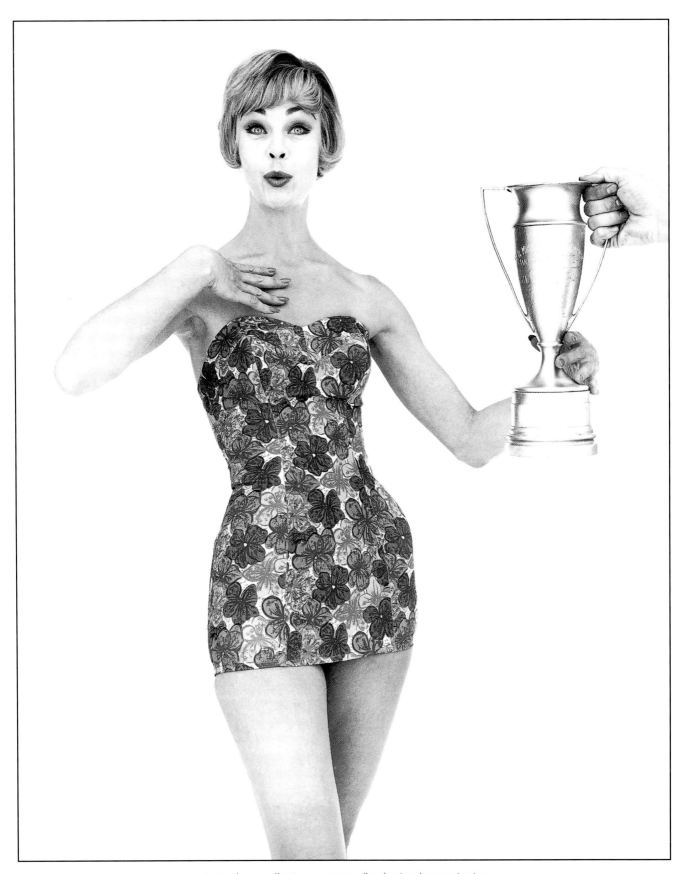

A strapless maillot in a summery floral print shows winning
style from the late 1950s. *Courtesy, Jimmy Mitchell.*

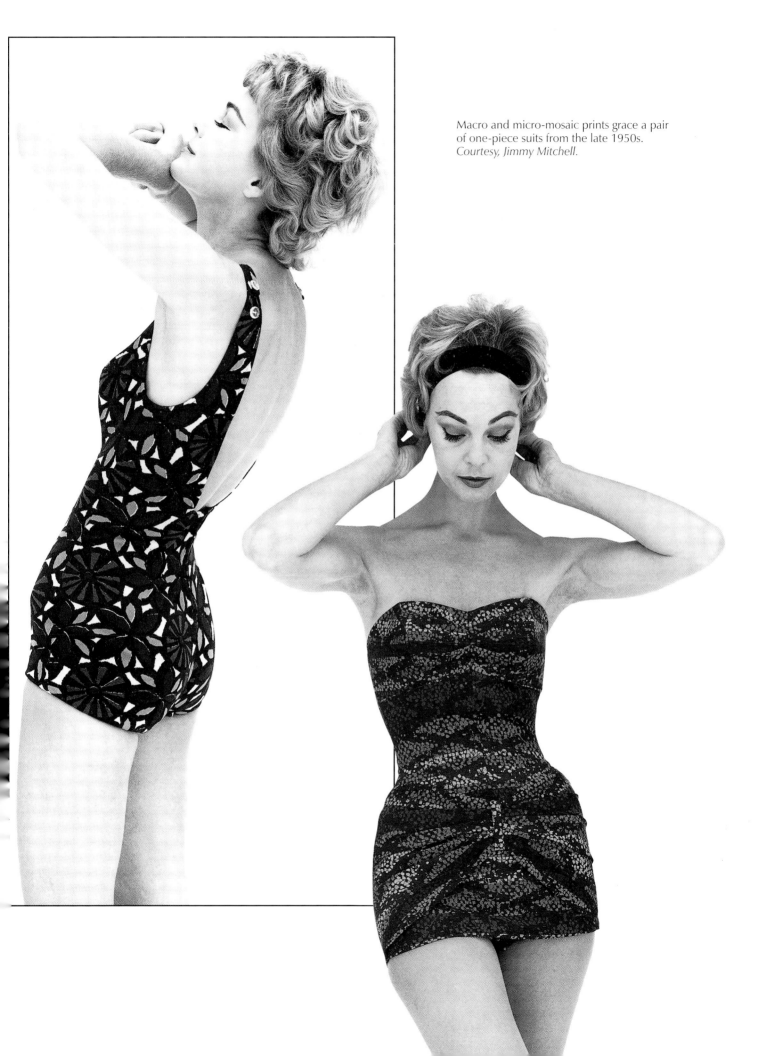

Macro and micro-mosaic prints grace a pair of one-piece suits from the late 1950s. *Courtesy, Jimmy Mitchell.*

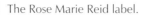
The Rose Marie Reid label.

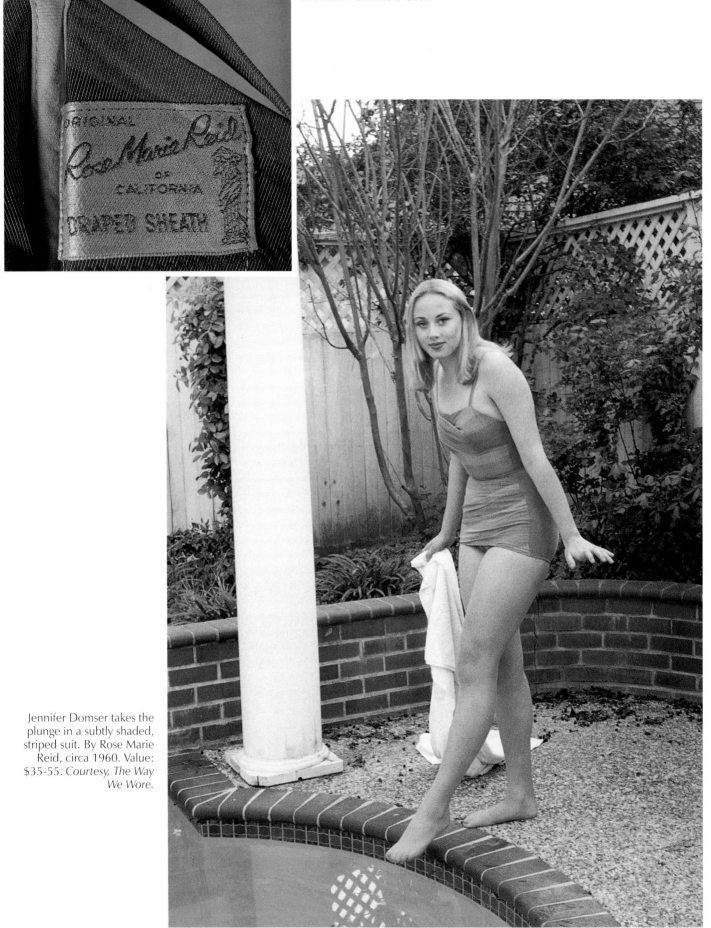

Jennifer Domser takes the plunge in a subtly shaded, striped suit. By Rose Marie Reid, circa 1960. Value: $35-55. *Courtesy, The Way We Wore.*

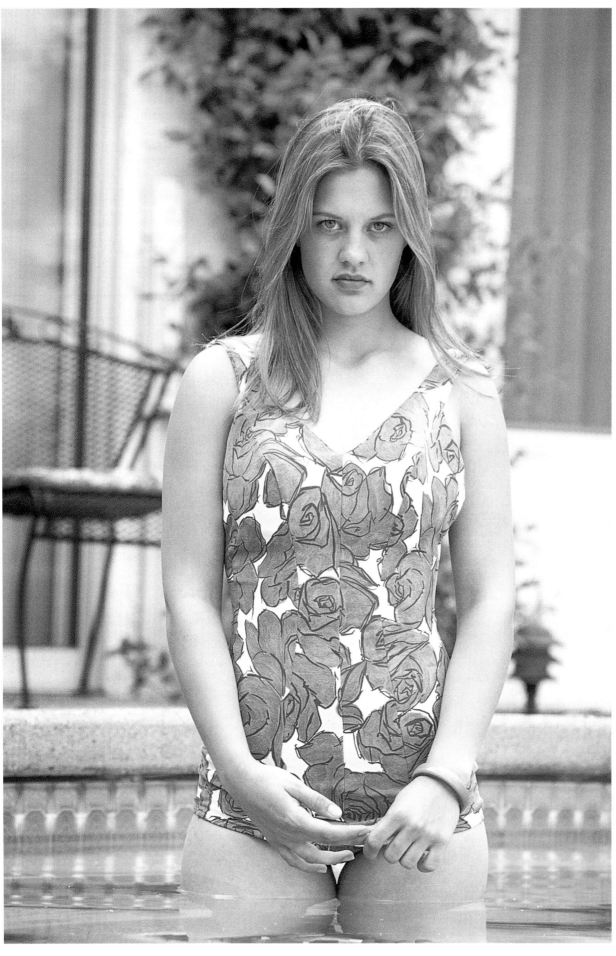

A bouquet of purple roses rising from the pool, on Angela D'Andrea. The suit is from Rose Marie Reid, circa 1965. Value: $25-35. *Courtesy, Luxe.*

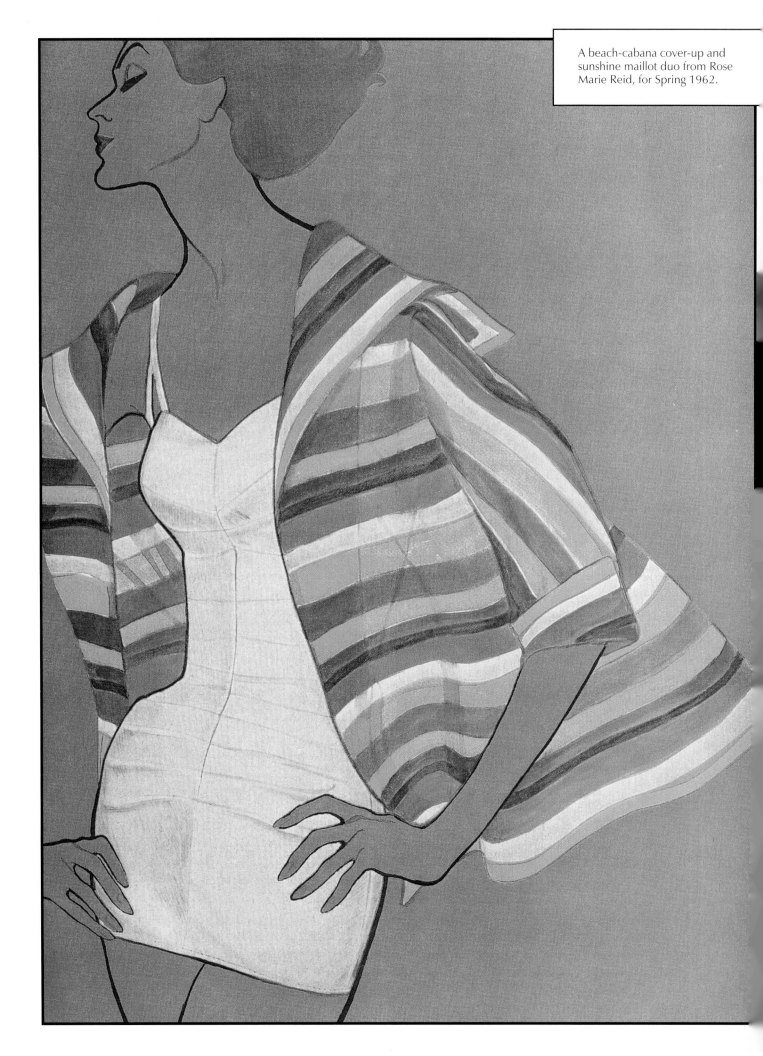

A beach-cabana cover-up and sunshine maillot duo from Rose Marie Reid, for Spring 1962.

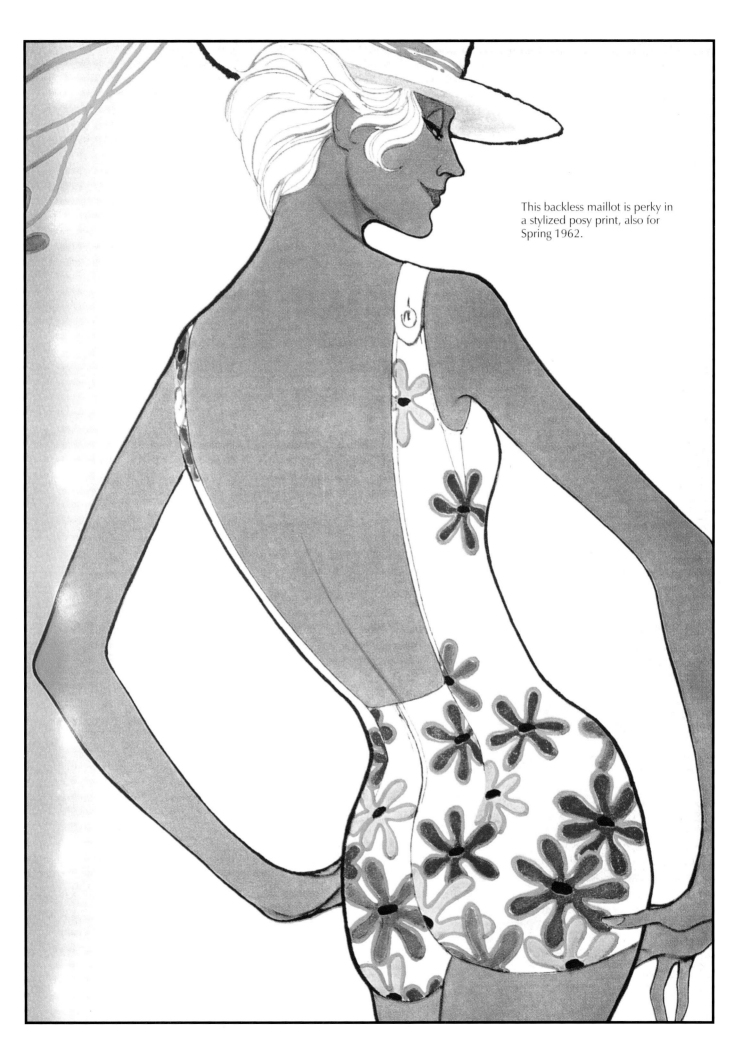

This backless maillot is perky in a stylized posy print, also for Spring 1962.

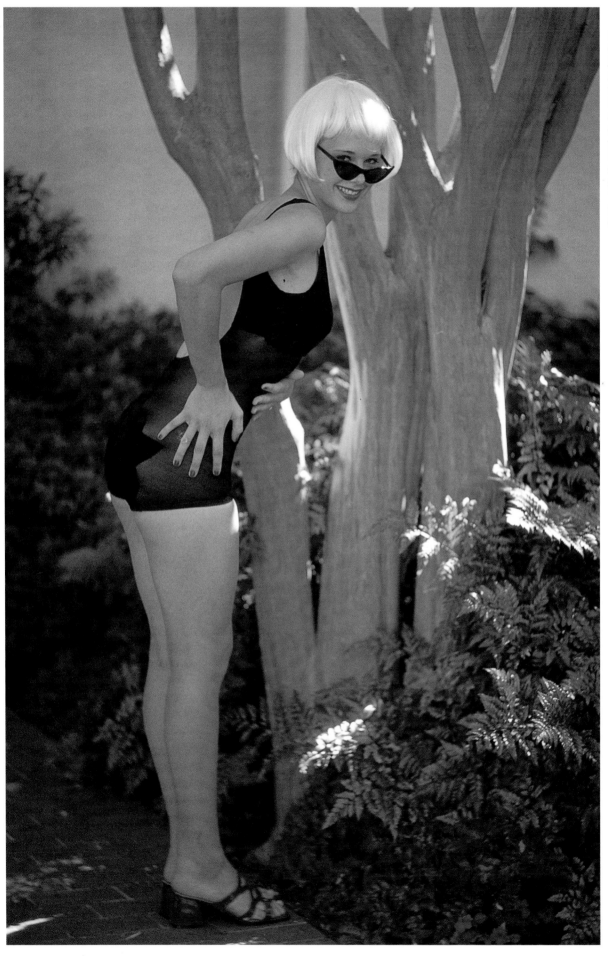

In the aftermath of Cole's mesh *Scandal Suit*, Rose Marie Reid offered this sexy sunbather in stretch velour and net. Nothing comes between you and your beach towel but a star-shaped swatch, circa 1965. Value: $75-95. *Courtesy, Cherry*.

Beach Party

A whole host of other influential swimwear companies made their corporate home in California. Here, a sampler of their winning beach styles.

Howard Greer

adapts the "MOLDED TORSO"*

of his

custom clothes

to

swimwear

by

Caltex

OF CALIFORNIA   NEW YORK ADDRESS: ROOM 307, HOTEL McALPIN

Noted Hollywood costumer and couturier Howard Greer designed for Caltex. This ad from November 1949 touted his *Molded Torso*.

Caltex

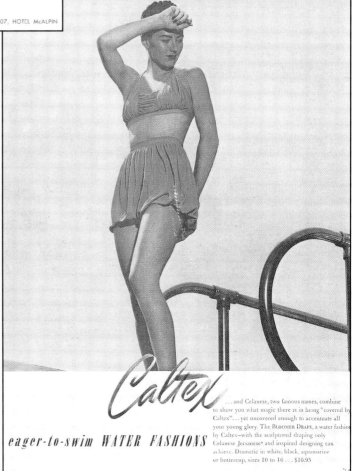

Early sarong styling was called the *Bloomer Drape* in this January 1946 ad by Caltex.

Caltex

eager-to-swim WATER FASHIONS

...and Celanese, two famous names, combine to show you what magic there is in being "covered by Caltex"...yet uncovered enough to accentuate all your young glory. The BLOOMER DRAPE, a water fashion by Caltex—with the sculptured draping only Celanese Jersanese* and inspired designing can achieve. Dramatic in white, black, aquamarine or buttercup, sizes 10 to 16 . . . $10.95

CALTEX OF CALIFORNIA · 2126 BEVERLY BOULEVARD · LOS ANGELES

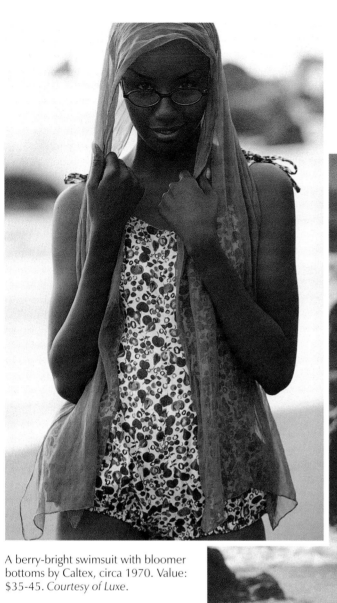

A berry-bright swimsuit with bloomer bottoms by Caltex, circa 1970. Value: $35-45. *Courtesy of Luxe.*

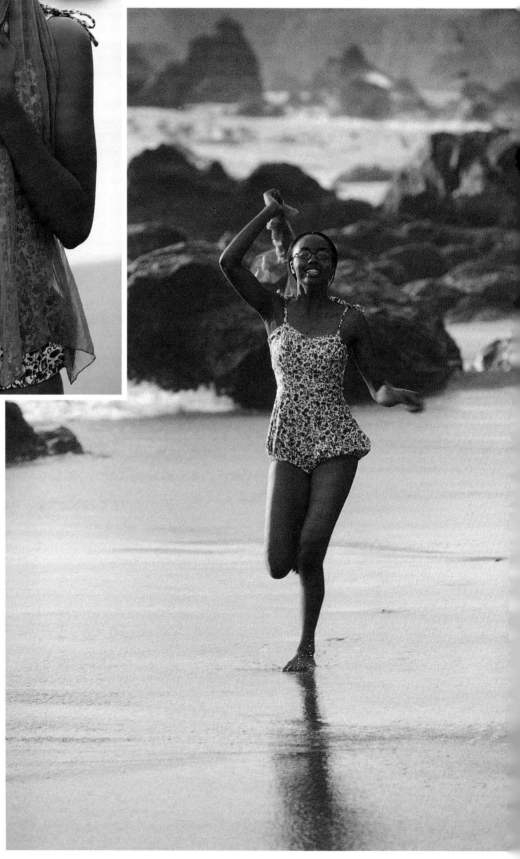

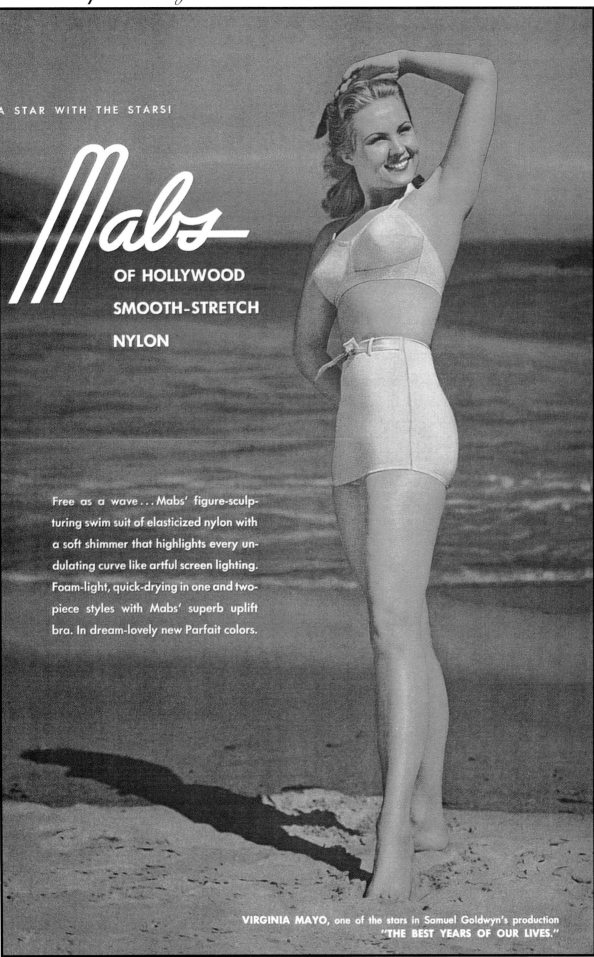

A STAR WITH THE STARS!

Mabs

OF HOLLYWOOD
SMOOTH-STRETCH
NYLON

Free as a wave . . . Mabs' figure-sculpturing swim suit of elasticized nylon with a soft shimmer that highlights every undulating curve like artful screen lighting. Foam-light, quick-drying in one and two-piece styles with Mabs' superb uplift bra. In dream-lovely new Parfait colors.

VIRGINIA MAYO, one of the stars in Samuel Goldwyn's production
"THE BEST YEARS OF OUR LIVES."

Mabs of Hollywood was modeled, fittingly, by actress Virginia Mayo in January 1947. This daring two-piece is elasticized nylon with a push-up "figure sculpting" bra.

Maurice Handler

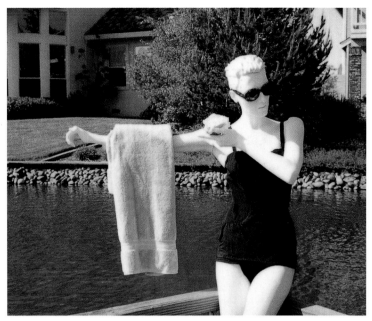

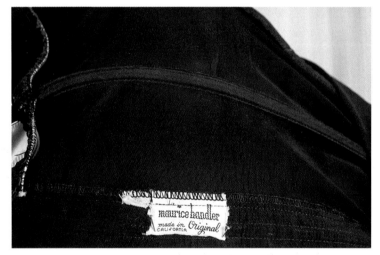

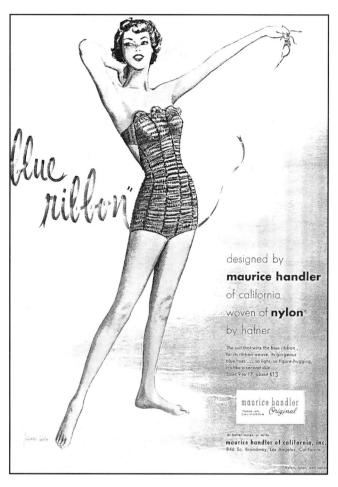

blue ribbon

designed by
maurice handler
of california
woven of **nylon***
by hafner

The suit that wins the blue ribbon . . .
for its ribbon weave, its gorgeous
blue hues . . . so light, so figure-hugging,
it's like a second skin . . .
Sizes 9 to 17, about $13

maurice handler
Original

At better stores, or write
maurice handler of california, inc.
846 So. Broadway, Los Angeles, California

Top left: Sunbathing, circa 1945. Value: $35-45. *Courtesy, The Way We Wore.*

Center left: The label is Maurice Handler.

Top right: High style from Maurice Handler of California. This Blue Ribbon suit was seamed from elasticized ribbon-weave cotton in 1953.

Marina del Mar

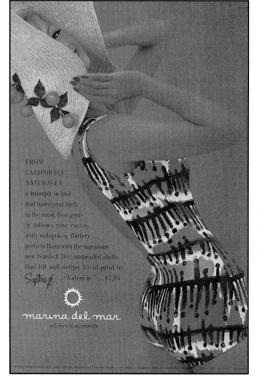

FROM
CALIFORNIA,
NATURALLY
a triumph in knit
that bares your back
to the waist, then gent-
ly follows your curves
with outspoken flattery . . .
perfects them with the ingenious
new Seashell Bra: suspended shells
that lift and define. Vivid print by
Saptra . . . "Valencia" . . . $17.95

marina del mar
california swimsuits

A stylized swimsuit in sunbelt colors, from Marina del Mar in January 1961. The company was promoting its *Seashell Bra*: " . . . suspended shells that lift and define."

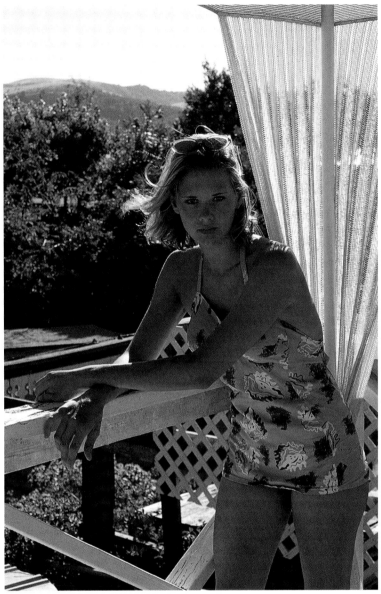

She sells seashells! This printed stretch cotton suit is typical of Marina del Mar, circa 1960. Value: $25-45. *Courtesy, Lottie Ballou.*

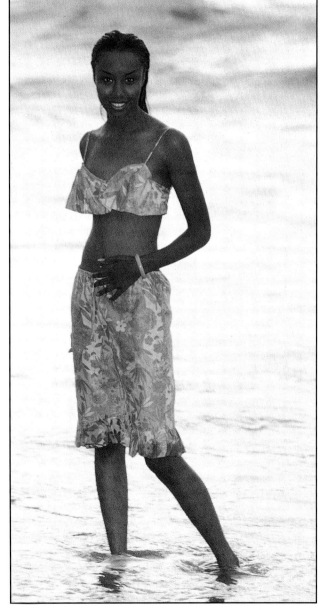

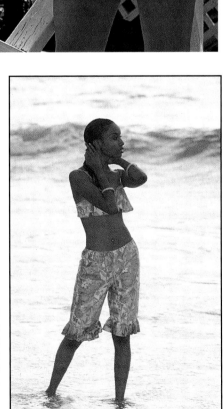

California Dreaming in a bikini top and jams, circa 1965. Tune in the transistor radio! The aptly-named label is "Beach Party." Value: $35-45. *Author's collection.*

chapter 3

POOL 'N PATIO

Activity was the sociopolitical catalyst that distinguished casual clothing, so favored by American women, from the stylized look cultivated by their European sisters. Reform dress was a necessity of the pioneer days, and by the Civil War there was a full-fledged movement for dress reform led by women who hoped to expand their lives beyond the kitchen and parlor.

> "Before there was an American fashion, there was an American style. It had its genesis in the patriotic determination, after the Revolutionary War, to wear homegrown, homespun, and home-sewn clothes, following the example of George and Martha Washington as well as such religious groups that had sought freedom in this country as the Amish and the Quakers. Relying on imported goods reflected poorly on America's independence, and ostentation in dress was viewed as epitomizing the rigidly delineated way of life under a monarchy. Simplicity in dress celebrated both self-sufficiency and the freedoms inherent in a democracy."
> —Caroline Rennolds Milbank, *New York Fashion*, 1989.

Remember Jo, the most active of the sisters in Louisa May Alcott's *Little Women?* In that fictional account of a New England family in the 1860s, Jo indulged in masculine pursuits like billiards and fencing. Such antics made her a favorite heroine, and a role model, for the girls of her day.

Jo liked to fence (verbally and physically) with the boys, in *Little Women*.

By the 1890s, reformists began to see their cause realized in the form of divided skirts and loosened corsets. Such clothing was much needed by woman who wanted to cross the gender divide from spectator sports to active sports. This "new woman" of a dawning century was epitomized in the drawings of Charles Dana Gibson.

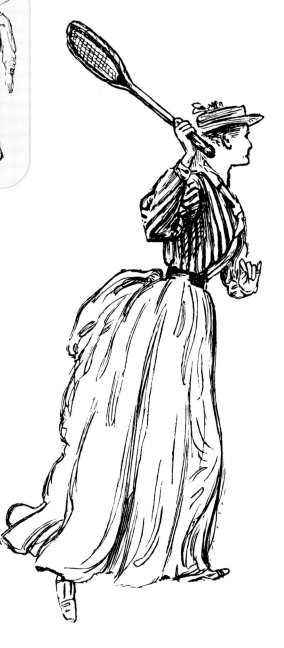

The Gibson Girl was athletic. She was usually shown in a simple boater, waist, and skirt.

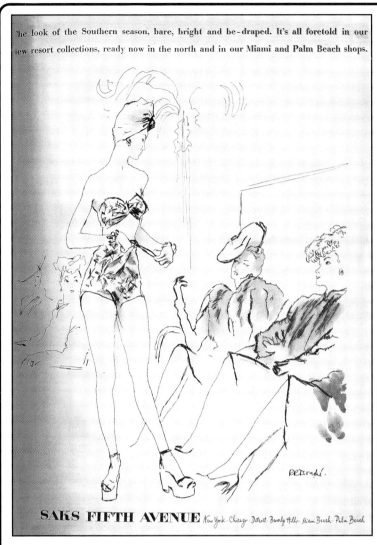

The look of the Southern season, bare, bright and be-draped. It's all foretold in our new resort collections, ready now in the north and in our Miami and Palm Beach shops.

SAKS FIFTH AVENUE New York · Chicago · Detroit · Beverly Hills · Miami Beach · Palm Beach

Resort styling in the salon as illustrated for Saks Fifth Avenue in the *Vogue* issue of January 1, 1945.

In the early 1900s, the great East Coast women's colleges made it socially acceptable to showcase brains *and* beauty with sensible dress styles. In the 1920s, the American flapper shed her corsets altogether and began demanding the freedom of slacks, shifts, and flat shoes for sporting and spectator-ing.

Although some European designers influenced the casual dress movement—especially Coco Chanel, with jersey separates for watching a polo match and loose pants for walking on a beach—the major contributions were made by American manufacturers who wholesaled affordable lines of pared-down French couture from their workshops on Seventh Avenue.

Great attention was paid to ordering the perfect resort wardrobe. This was true for the socialites who flew pre jet-set to Cannes and Cancun, to those who only packed for a weekend at the shore.

It was during World War II, after the German occupation of Paris and the stoppage of fashion exports, that American designers were finally recognized. History would show that, as a group, their greatest contribution was in separates. The concept of creating a coordinated line of casual clothing that could be "mixed 'n matched" by the consumer is uniquely American, and something the sports-minded California designers particularly excelled at.

"The fashion that L-85 built." This cartoon explains how American designers rose to the fabric shortage occasion, as seen in *Vogue* on February 1, 1944.

The fashion that L-85 built

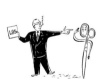

This is the Man (Donald Nelson)
who made the rule
that sent Design
to a strict new school.

This is the Skirt
and these the Shears
that narrow the line
to lean war years.

This is the Tunic
that's smooth over hips
that are cased in skirts
that are close as slips

This is the Jacket
that's boxy and square
that tops the tight skirts
that all of us wear.

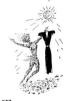

This is the Cap Sleeve
next summer will bring;
it's best above skirts
that are slim as a string.

This is the Coat
that's belted and shorn
that always looks better
when tight skirts are worn.

Separated geographically from New York City, which became even more of a focal point for the garment industry in the war years, California designers found it difficult to gain the recognition of major department store buyers. That all changed in the 1942, not only by reason of the blackout of Paris, but also because that's the year Adrian quit his job as the head of costume design for Metro-Goldwyn-Mayer to open his own salon in Beverly Hills.

For a decade, women across America had dreamed of dressing in the same fabulous clothes that Adrian designed for luminous MGM stars like Jean Harlow, Greta Garbo, and Joan Crawford—now they could. Once he began marketing ready-to-wear, the demand was so great that the privileged stores with contracts to sell "Adrian Originals" had to ration his crisp suits and flowing gowns, one or two to the customer.

That kind of sales power commanded the attention of buyers, who flocked from New York to place their orders at his three seasonal showings. There was always a preview fashion show for the buyers and press, but the buyers could only meet Adrian in person by appointment. They filled in their calendars by making the circuit of other couturiers, like the young James Galanos. Along the way, they also visited the many sportswear houses sprouting up in Los Angeles.

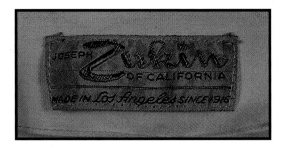

The label for Joe Zukin of Los Angeles, an early sportswear house.

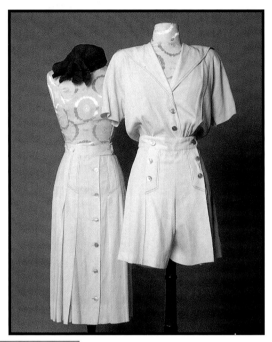

These separates in white sharkskin are meticulously tailored—a fine example of 1940s sportstyle.

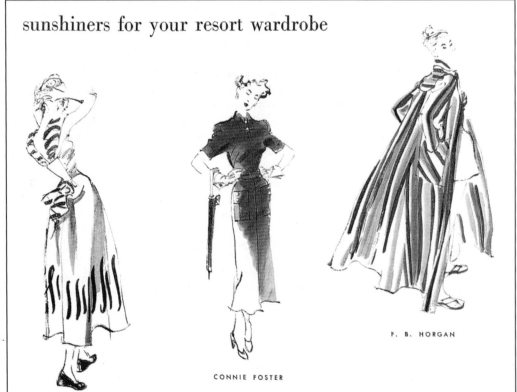

sunshiners for your resort wardrobe

FAY FOSTER

CONNIE FOSTER

F. B. HORGAN

"Sunshiners for your resort wardrobe." This bright parade was offered by the California firms Fay Foster, Connie Foster, and F.B. Horgan, in 1945.

126

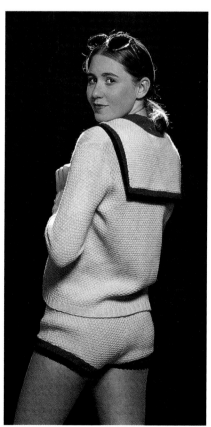

San Francisco's Apparel City

Apparel City was dubbed a "World of Tomorrow" by the local newspapers.

"Working conditions hit a new high. Modern buildings, radiant with sunshine and fresh air, are already reported to have contributed to raising the level of production."—*San Francisco News*, 1947.

This apron sundress with matching stole pairs chic with comfort. From Lanz of California for Spring 1957, in pastel Caliente Cloth with black braid trim.

The garment manufacturers headquartered in San Francisco benefited as well from the demand for consumer goods in the war years.

Both Koret of California, Inc. and Alice of California were founded in San Francisco—the city that was by then affectionately nicknamed "Paris of the West" by reason of its reputation for style and sophistication—and both saw their sales volume skyrocket in the years following the attack on Pearl Harbor. Shortly after the war ended, Koret and Alice, along with about thirty other garment manufacturers from Northern California, set up shop in Apparel City. This was a brand-new industrial park that rose from a wartime trailer camp in the Potrero District.

In 1947, Koret and Alice joined other Apparel City manufacturers in a "San Francisco to Paris" fashion show orchestrated by the local Manufacturers & Wholesalers Association under the leadership of Adolph Schumann, founder of the Lilli Ann coat and suit house.

Schumann and the others realized how desperate postwar Europe was for mass-produced goods, including clothing. Even so, according to the *San Francisco News,* there were initial misgivings about taking fashions to France: "Thirty-three manufacturers risked being laughed at by the French. The nerve of showing American apparel that wives, coeds and stenographers can buy for $15 to $79, when Paris designs styles to sell to the elite few at an average cost said to be $600 a garment."

Happily, when the verdict was in and the sales orders were tallied, the show was judged a success. "Paris couturiers and the public were amazed that [Americans] could mass-produce such clothes within the reach of the average purse," the *News* glowed.

These knit separates trimmed in red and blue were made by Koret of California in the 1940s. Value: Special. *Courtesy, The Way We Wore.*

Unfortunately, finding vintage casual clothing is difficult, since it tended to be worn out by the original owners. Sometimes, a cache of dead stock or sample goods will appear on the market, as was the case when Koret sold its warehouse inventory about ten years ago.

Along with the casual clothing labels, there were many other California companies that would be worthy of inclusion in a vintage collection, such as Graff, Gantner, Trude, Connie Foster, Rough Rider, Fleischmann, Strawberry Patch, California Girl, and Campus Casuals.

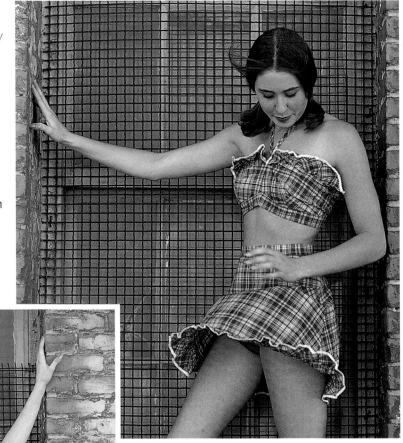

Two views of a two-piece rayon playset from the 1940s (no label). In case of a breeze, red shorts were attached to the trapeze skirt. Value: $55-75. *Courtesy, Luxe.*

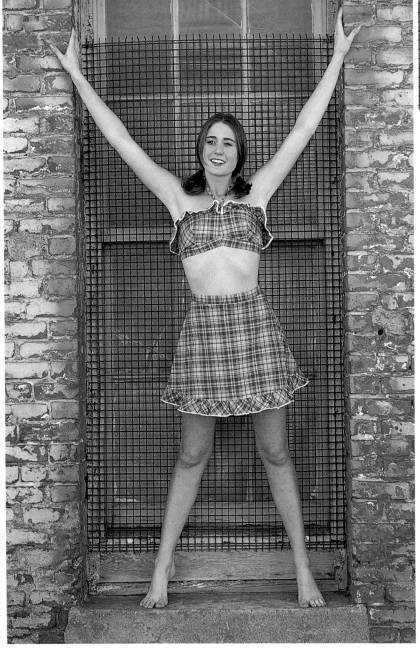

Koret

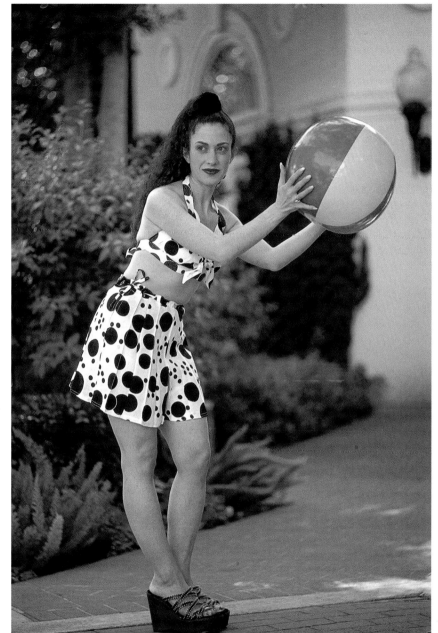

The husband-and-wife team of Stephanie and Joe Koret founded a business on skirts. It was she who thought of top-stitching pleated skirts to fold flat and hold their shape; she also used a drawstring waist that adjusted to a variety of sizes. It was he who had the background in wholesaling and knew how to get the skirts mass-produced and marketed.

Stephanie had studied design at San Francisco's Fashion Art School before marrying Joe and joining him on his traveling sales route. For many years, they carried a line of wholesale sportswear and sweaters, which she occasionally modeled. Traveling throughout eleven Western states, they learned what items were in demand.

In 1938, their customers began urging the Korets to offer skirts that would match their line of sweaters. That's when Stephanie put her schooling to good use, designing the *Trikskirt*.

This early separates set, in Dalmatian-dot linen, features *Trikskirt* pleating. Value: $75-95. *Courtesy, It's About Time.*

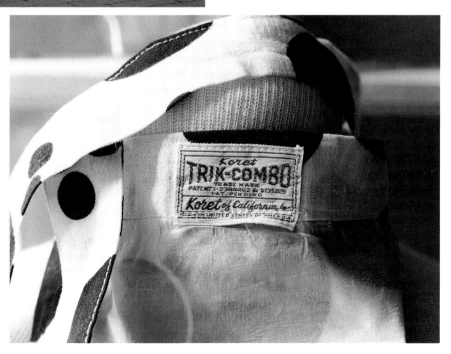

The patented trademark is *Trik-Combo.*

129

Having patented Stephanie's design, the Korets incorporated in September 1939. Their first year in business resulted in a disappointing sales volume of only $20,000. Then they advertised nationally, and women began snapping up those tricky skirts. By 1941, Koret, Inc. passed the million-dollar mark in annual sales.

The company continued to grow rapidly, especially after Stephanie improved her original design with a process for permanent pleating, under the label *Pleetskirt*. Her process called for heating batches of one hundred skirts at a time in a steam oven, thereby baking in the pleats. The pleats were guaranteed to stay in place for six months and remain crisp for the life of the skirt with pressing.

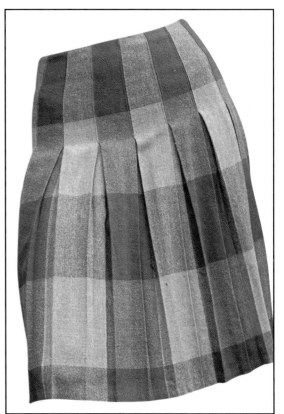

Pleats all around, baked in and stitched down.

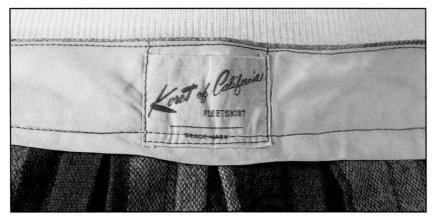

The *Pleetskirt*.

Stephanie's ingenuity didn't stop there; a few years later, she and Joe were patenting her *Girdlslax* and *Slim Hip Slax* designs. These slacks featured a specially-cut crotch and waistband to solve the problem of baggy bottoms and flapping shirt-tails.

Along with a host of other garment manufacturers, the Korets were headquartered in new facilities at Apparel City, on the outskirts of San Francisco. Their 1946 books showed an international business with $12 million in annual sales. Eventually, the Korets opened regional offices and showrooms in Los Angeles, Honolulu, Atlanta, Chicago, and New York.

This was a full sportswear line with all manner of skirts, slacks, blouses, sweaters, jackets dresses, beachwear, and sportswear. An early ad slogan boasted: "Sportswear Created From Life in the Sun." As their business grew, the Korets diversified into suits, jackets, and even handbags, but always with an emphasis on casual California style.

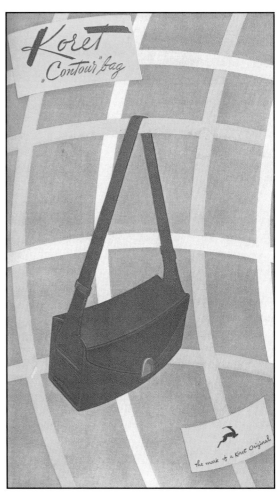

The sporty *Contour* bag was advertised by Koret in 1945.

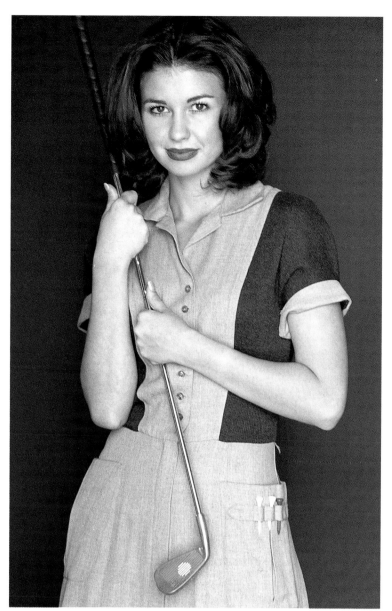

A golfer, with tee-ties at the belt and other sporty detailing (circa 1940). It's worn with great verve by Julie Durda. Value: Special. *Courtesy, The Way We Wore.*

The Korets used only union labor with an emphasis on quality. Stephanie personally inspected all samples, and they could not be produced without her signature on the label. Buttonholes were hand-finished, collars had sweatbands, pockets had plackets, seams were a half-inch and whip-finished, and hems were three inches deep or handkerchief-rolled.

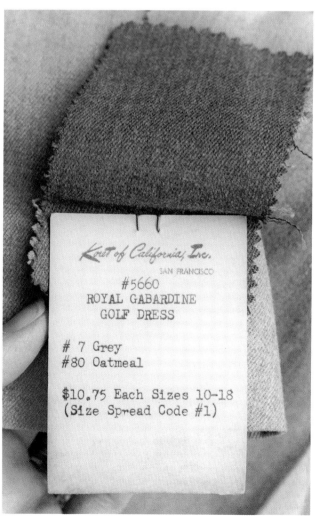

This dress, an unsold sample, still bears the original salesman's hangtag with fabric swatches of Royal Gabardine in grey and oatmeal.

To ensure reliability of the Koret label, thousands of garments were removed from mainstream distribution and sold at discount, or donated to charity. "It may seem trite to say, but if we have the least doubt on a garment meeting rigid quality controls or of a customer being dissatisfied, we mark that garment in heavy black ink across the label, *Seconds*." So explained Joe Koret to the *San Francisco News* in 1946.

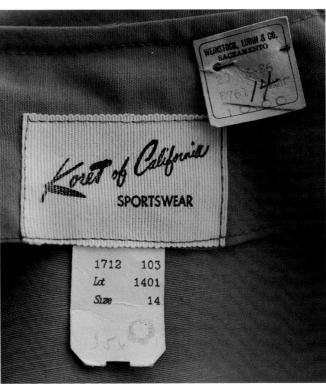

According to the label, this is a size 14; by today's standards, it would be an 8.

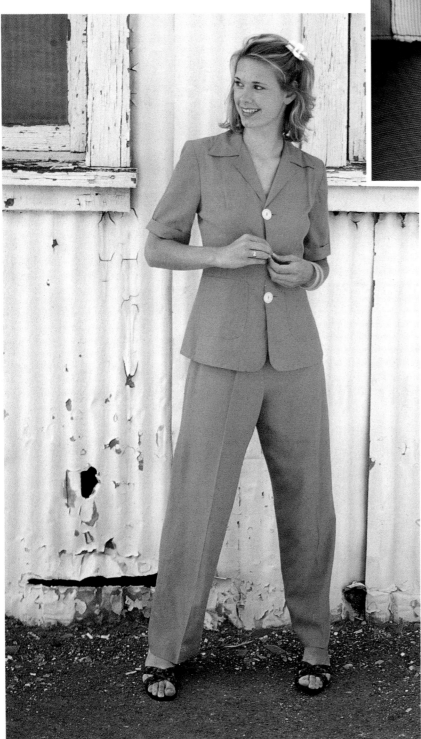

Elizabeth Haskett shows a tangy two-piece pant set, perfect for weekends in the 1940s or today. Value: $45-75. *Courtesy, Cheap Thrills.*

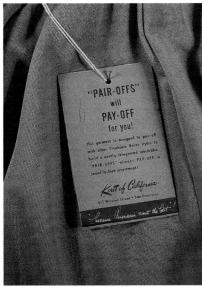

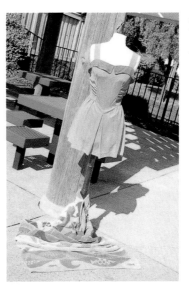

Top: The one-piece playsuit shown at right was part of Koret's *Pair Offs* line of separates, and was probably matched to a coordinated skirt.

Center & bottom: The original hangtag and label for the playsuit.

An orange skarkskin playsuit with rhinestone trim, another unsold sample (circa 1945). Value: Special. *Courtesy, The Way We Wore.*

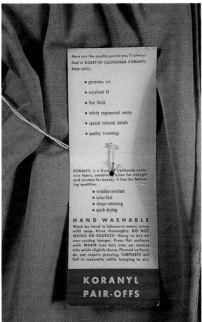

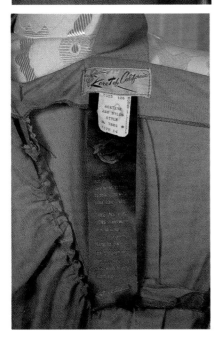

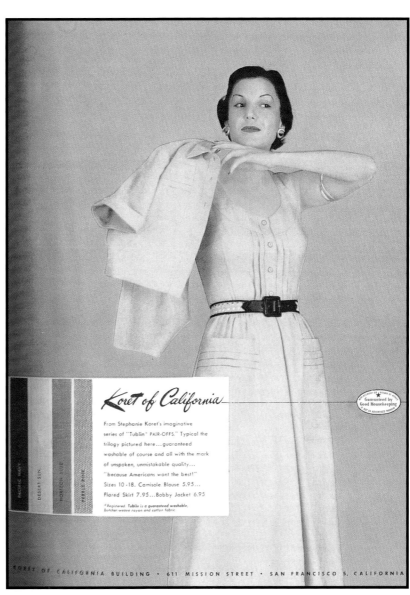

This set (camisole, skirt, and bolero) is from the *Pair Offs* collection in 1951. It was available in a rainbow of rayon-blend colors.

Stephanie's gift for picking fabrics was as much a part of the company's success as the originality of her designs. She selected sunny printed cotton and linen in the 1940s and 1950s, doubleknit and polyester in the 1960s and 1970s. These fabrics came from the best names in the business, such as Hoffman, Cone, Enka, and Klopman. As befits a sportswear house, all fabrics were chosen with an eye toward packing ease and wash 'n wearability.

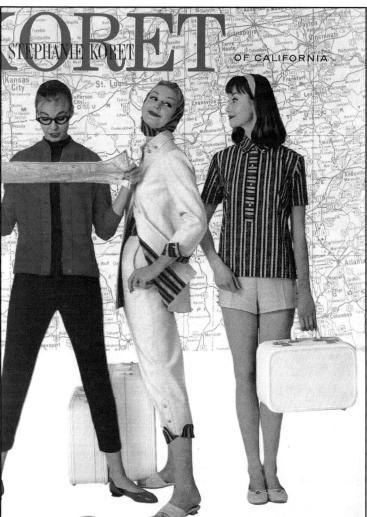

Vacation togs from Koret, for Resort 1957.

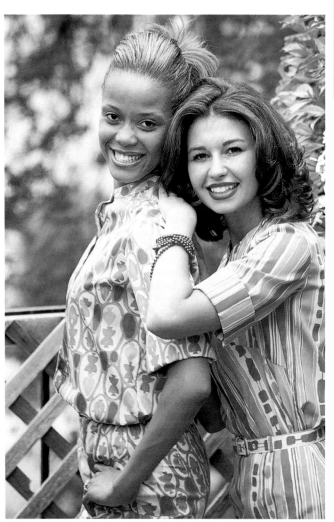

In the 1950s, the company began to specialize in coordinated clothing sold as separates or three-piece sets. Long vests, simple shells, long and short skirts, slacks, shorts, and culottes were typical mix 'n match pieces. These were cut from the same printed fabric with coordinated buttons and trim.

Stephanie Koret often ordered fabric in different colorways. Shown on Vesha and Julie, a two-piece shirtwaist in shades of melon or nutmeg with the punch of lemon. Value each: $55-75. *Courtesy, The Way We Wore.*

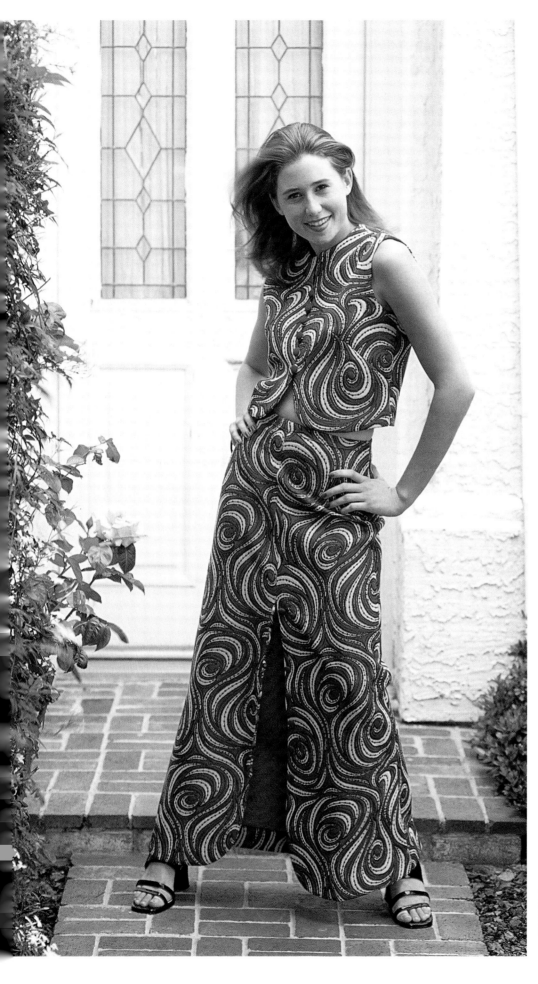

The company flourished through the 1970s, always keeping abreast of the newest trends in casual wear, like this mod maxi-skirt and vest.

Kim Davidson is mod to party in a two-piece doubleknit, shown *sans* blouse. Value: $75-95. *Courtesy, The Way We Wore*.

Elizabeth Haskett thinks summertime in a pink chambray playset, circa 1965 (bandeau added). Value: $35-55. *Courtesy, The Way We Wore.*

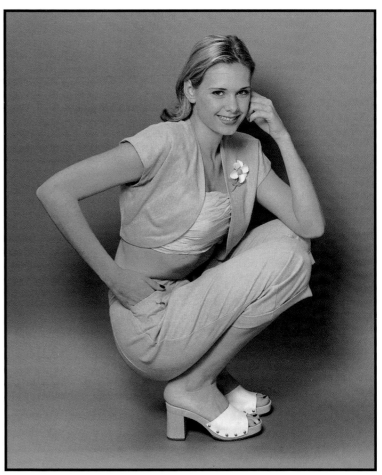

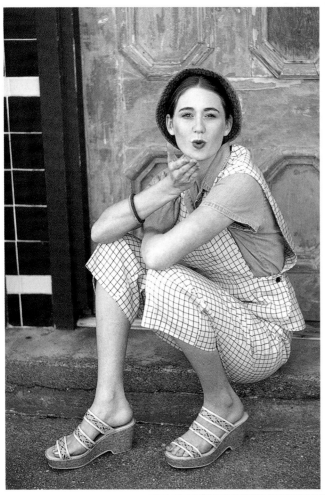

Kim is looking sweet and sassy in a jerkin and Capris checked red, cream, and blueberry, circa 1950 (blouse and hat not vintage). Value: $55-65. *Courtesy, The Way We Wore.*

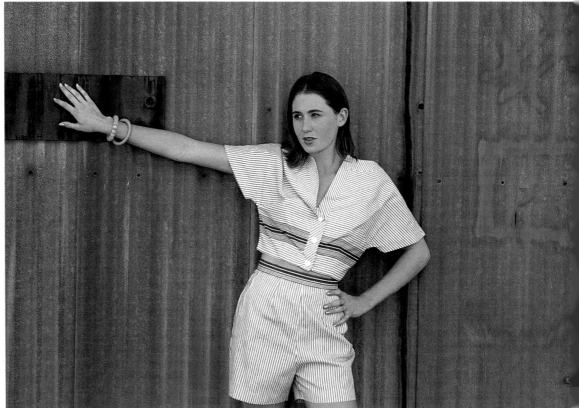

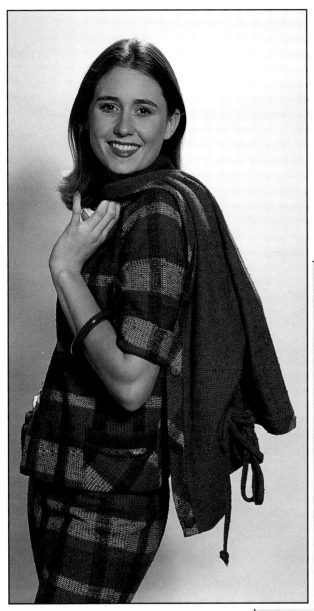

A three-piece weekender in slubby
rust and bark plaid. Value: $95-125.
Courtesy, The Way We Wore.

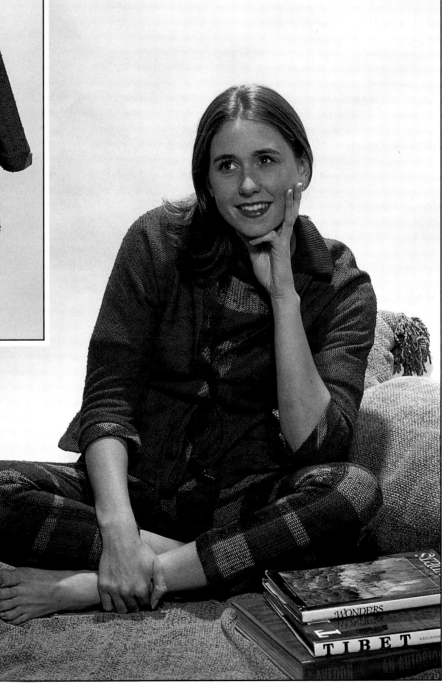

Opposite page
Bottom: A shorts set in atypical fall tones.
The horizontal stripes give this casual outfit
great flair. Value: $55-65. *Courtesy, The*
Way We Wore.

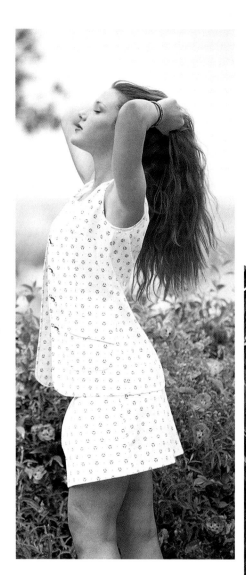

Three easy pieces for golf or tennis in the mid-1960s. The shell is cotton jersey; the shorts and vest are sailcloth. All are shown in a brown-on-white print, on Angela Prichard. Value: $55-75. *Courtesy, The Way We Wore.*

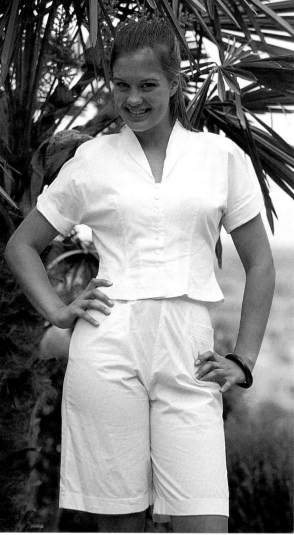

Angela D'Andrea sports a white pique Bermuda short set, circa 1960. Value: $55-75. *Courtesy, The Way We Wore.*

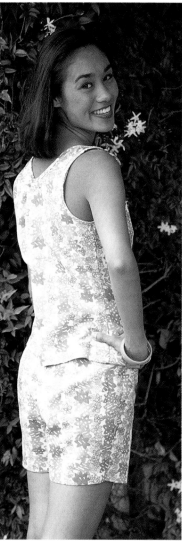

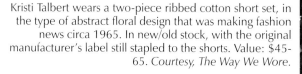

Kristi Talbert wears a two-piece ribbed cotton short set, in the type of abstract floral design that was making fashion news circa 1965. In new/old stock, with the original manufacturer's label still stapled to the shorts. Value: $45-65. *Courtesy, The Way We Wore.*

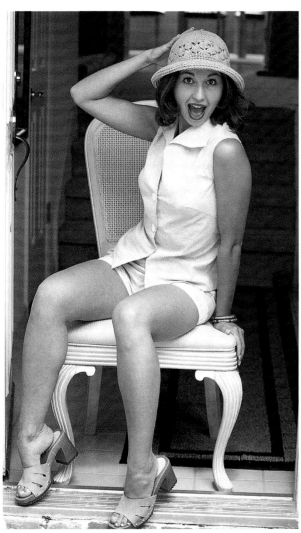

This seersucker set came with a choice of lace-trimmed shorts or culottes (not shown), circa 1960. Value: $45-55. *Courtesy, The Way We Wore.*

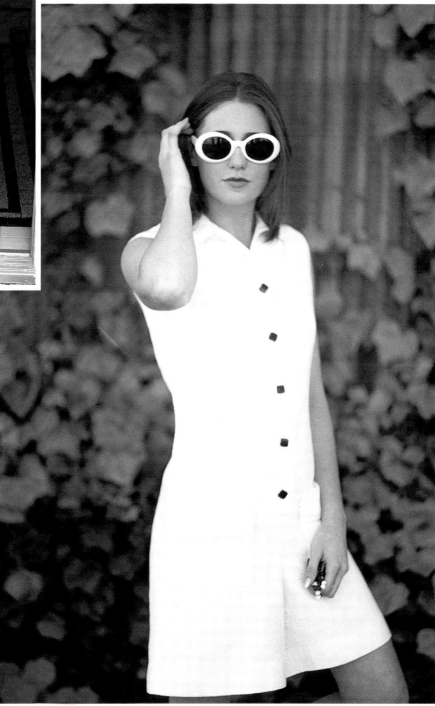

You could serve tennis, or drinks, in this short jumper, circa 1965. The crisp white pique plays against black buttons. Value: $45-65. *Courtesy, The Way We Wore.*

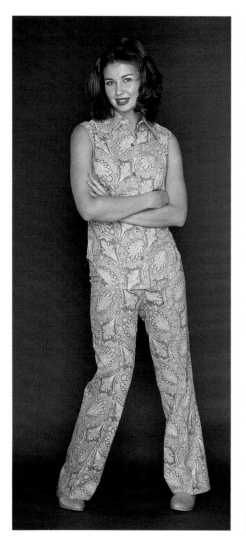

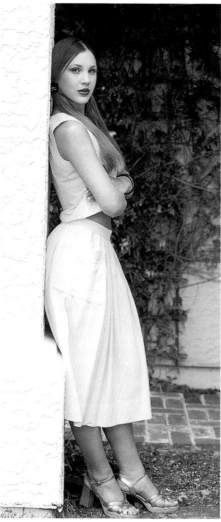

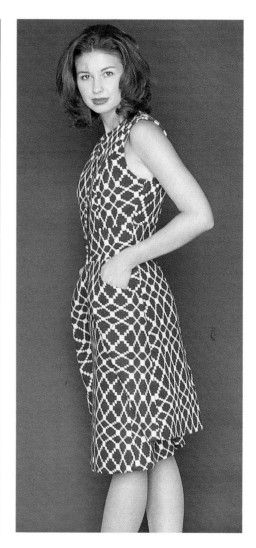

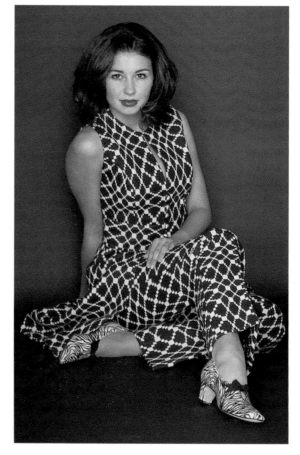

Top left: The with-it pants set in a sophisticated paisley linen. It was also offered as a skirt set in the same print, different colorway, circa 1970. Value: $55-75. *Courtesy, The Way We Wore.*

Top center: Angela Prichard is jaunty in jonquil rayon with the look of sharkskin, circa 1955. The vest, with its quilt detailing, was meant to be worn over a blouse. Value: $55-75. *Courtesy, The Way We Wore.*

Top right & bottom: Brown and white houndstooth is groovy for a vest-and-pants suit from the late 1960s. The only problem Julie Durda has is choosing between the skirt or bell bottoms from this coordinated separates set. Value: $75-125. *Courtesy, The Way We Wore.*

Alice of California

It's a story of rags to riches. Or in this case, rags to rag trade. The true adventures of Krist Gunderson, who founded Alice of California in 1925, seem like the fictionalized account of Horatio Algier.

Gunderson was orphaned in Iceland at the age of six and earned his own way in life from that point forward, being indentured to a farmer. He learned to read, but had no formal schooling. While still a teenager, he was apprenticed to the owner of a fishing boat and sailed the Arctic Ocean for three years. Then Gunderson managed to "jump ship" and escape to Norway, where he sold books door-to-door.

By 1904, he had earned his own passage to America and gladly immigrated. When Gunderson's ship sailed into the harbor at Ellis Island, he was just twenty-one years old and frail of build. After paying the ferry passage to New York City, Gunderson had a dime to his name—he spent that on a loaf of bread, which he lived on for three days until he had a job.

Eager to start a new life in the land of opportunity, Gunderson was handicapped by his lack of education and scant command of English. After learning rudimentary English in night school at the YMCA, he took various jobs and started a family. With his wife and three children, he eventually trekked west, finding work in the stockroom of a wholesale drygoods house in Portland, Oregon.

The pay was meager, just $15 a week—not enough to support a family, even in the early 1920s. When Gunderson asked for a raise, his boss said that was all a stockboy was worth: "The trouble with you, Krist, is you're working from your neck down. Work with your head, and you'll be worth more."

That's when Gunderson remembered his success as a door-to-door salesman, and convinced the wholesaler to let him peddle "dead stock" from the warehouse on the road. He was so successful that his income soared from $15 a week, to $900 and even $1500 a month.

The Gundersons moved to Los Angeles in search of greener pastures and found them in sales for a local dress manufacturer. Buoyed by this success, but determined to make it really big, Gunderson started his own dress business with a $1500 loan. It was 1925 when he launched the Lady Alice line of casual dresses, slacks and blouses. The Lil' Alice junior line was added soon after.

Krist Gunderson in the mid-1940s.

Lil' Alice
STITCHED AND STYLED
IN CALIFORNIA

"YUM-YUM" by Lil' Alice. Shades of the Mikado. Flirtatious rayon fan print that's perfect for Sunday in the Park, or a week end in the country.

The *Yum-Yum* was an early daytimer by Lil' Alice, as advertised in 1947.

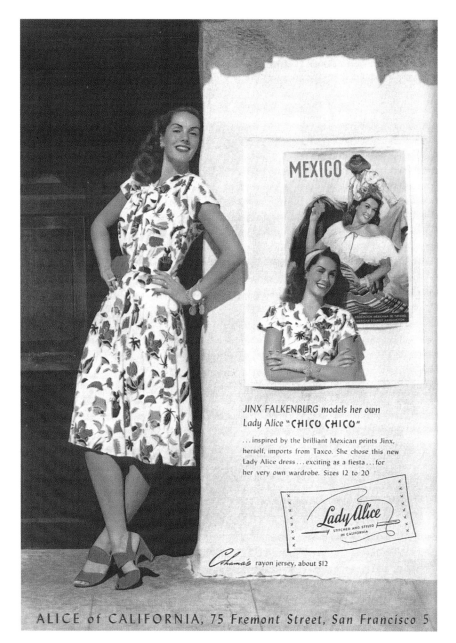

The *Chico Chico* in rayon jersey was shown in 1946 on Jinx Falkenburg, a radio talk show host and one of the supermodels of her day. The suggested retail price for this south-of-the border dress was $12.

B y the 1930s, the company had an annual sales volume of $150,000 and by the 1940s it had shot to $1,000,000. In 1947, Alice established a four-story factory at the new industrial park in San Francisco, Apparel City.

Gunderson's son Harold followed in his father's footsteps, working his way up from stock clerk to Vice President. It was Harold who worked closely with the design staff, to keep the company's lines relevant for consumers.

Starting about 1930, Carolyn Perena became the head designer at Alice. As profiled by the *California Stylist* in July 1967, she defined a fresh resort look, marked by her love of exotic prints and her allegiance to four basic standards: "Colorful, casual, comfortable and *Californian.*"

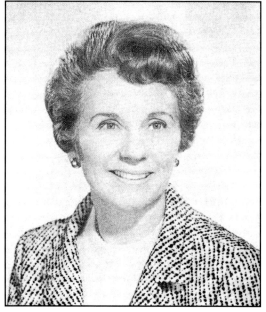

Carolyn Perena, head designer.

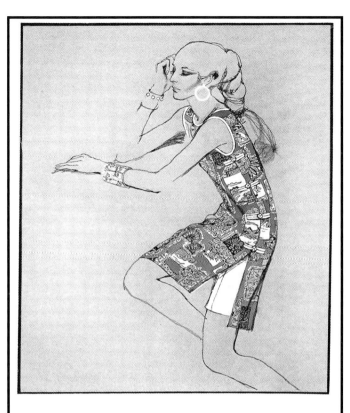

print and plain

. . . meet in a two part "Tea Timer" set in imported hand-screened cotton with perma-press finish. Dramatic at-home style #14318, in sizes 8-16, retails under $30. In combinations of green, orange or blue. S.F.: 60 Dorman Ave.; L.A.: 110 E. 9th St.; N.Y.: 1407 Broadway. BY ALICE

by alice

Exotic Sixties styles from Alice of California. The *Tea Timer* tunic and the dramatic *Kimono* were cut from imported hand-screened cotton.

B y the 1960s, Perena and the Gundersons had dropped the Lady Alice and Lil' Alice labels to establish three distinct new lines. They were Alice, with casual and career-girl looks; Krist, for date and special occasion styles; and Alice Polynesian, for weekend and loungewear.

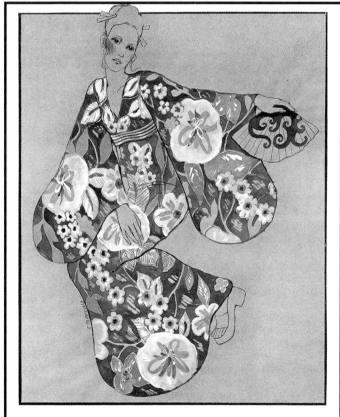

kimono creation

. . . a dramatically oriental treatment of sleeve and screening brings out the far eastern influence in a lounger of hand screened cotton satin with a perma-press finish. Style 14270 is available in Petite, Small, Medium or Large, in predominantly green, pink or purple combinations.

| SAN FRANCISCO: 60 Dorman Ave. | LOS ANGELES: 110 E. 9th St. Suite 333 | MIAMI: Merchandise Mart, Suite 2243 | DALLAS: Apparel Mart Suite 1316 | ATLANTA: Merchandise Mart Suite 4J-11 |

by alice

"The Gundersons and Carolyn work in perfect unison [as] one of the strongest teams in California fashion, proof that happiness and success don't kill creativity," according to the *Stylist*. "Their success formula is traditional with the firm: modestly priced dresses in key with the times."

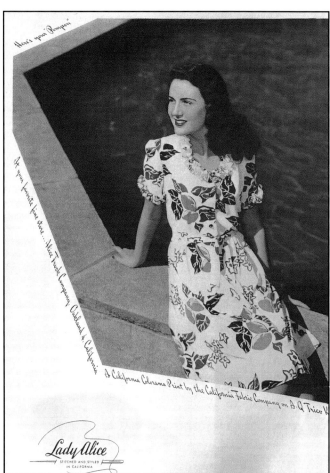

This bold floral *Pompon* sundress with ruffle detail was in keeping with the mood of 1945.

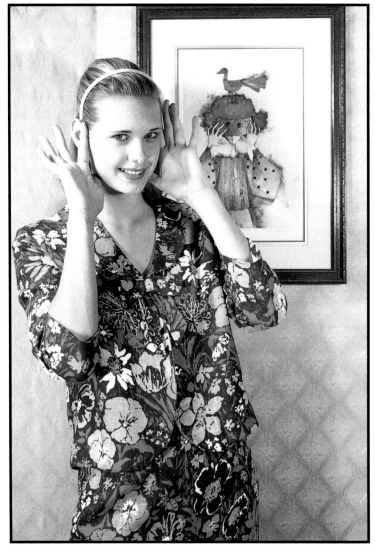

In 1965, make it an even bolder floral pattern on a little luncheon suit.

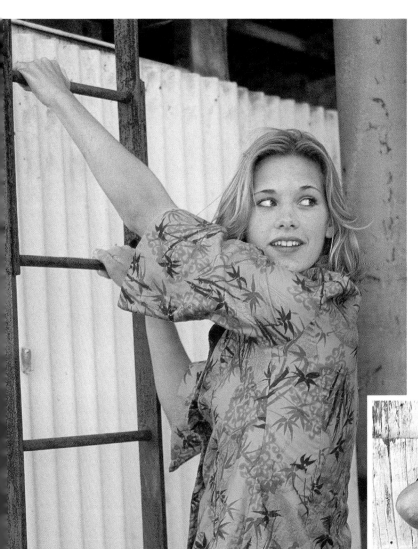

Elizabeth Haskett escapes the ordinary in a print pantsuit that's cut like pajamas (circa 1965). The label is Alice Polynesian. Value: $45-65. *Courtesy, It's About Time.*

plaid 'n' pretty

Alice of California advertised a relatively conservative A-line in November 1967.

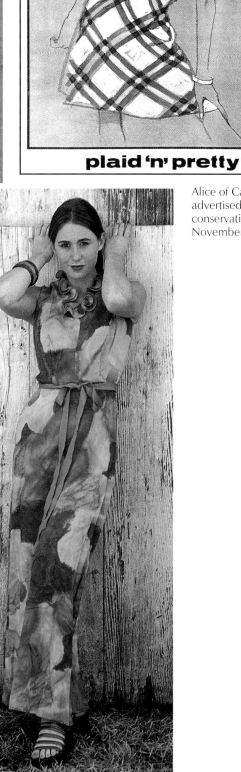

Kim Davidson puts on the charm in a hostess gown, a tropical print by Alice Polynesian (circa 1975). Value: $25-35. *Author's collection.*

145

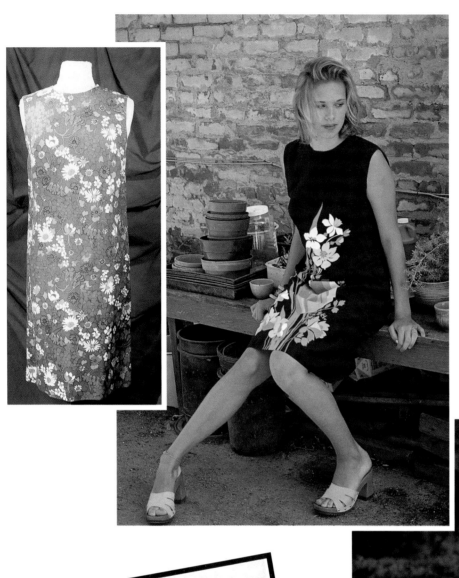

Two cotton shifts in floral prints by Alice of California, circa 1965.

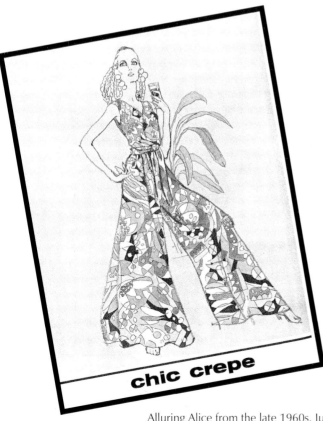

chic crepe

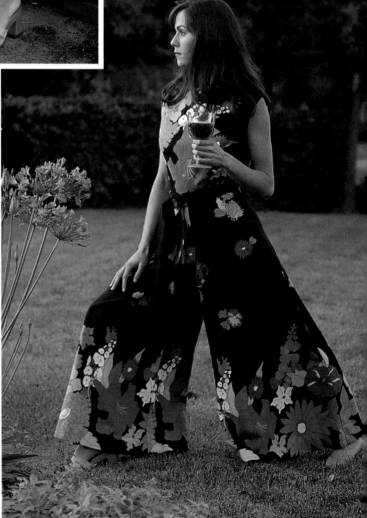

Alluring Alice from the late 1960s. Just look at the size of those bell-bottoms!

Lanz

The label sometimes read Lanz of Salzburg, but that only reflected the ethnic origins of company founder Sepp Lanz. In fact it was Lanz of California, as made in Los Angeles and distributed on both coasts.

The company retained his name even after Sepp sold his one-third interest in 1951. Soon after, he and wife Denise Lanz founded Denise Designs, again in Los Angeles. She was installed as head designer for the new company, using the same style principles that had made Lanz so refreshing for the junior market: white collars, lace trim, and crisp cotton fabrics often trimmed with a touch of Alpine charm like embroidered ribbons.

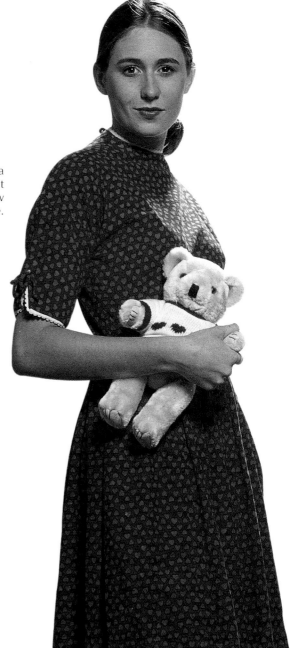

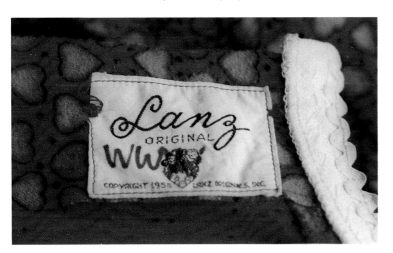

Jimmy Mitchell models an early 1950s charmer from Lanz. *Courtesy, Jimmy Mitchell.*

The archetypical Lanz dress. It's pretty and demure with a jewel neckline and bow-tied sleeves, in a heart-print flannel trimmed with white rickrack. (The skirt falls below the knees.) Value: $55-75. *Courtesy, The Way We Wore.*

The Lanz label, bearing a copyright date of 1958. There was also a Lanz of Austria label, from the same parent company.

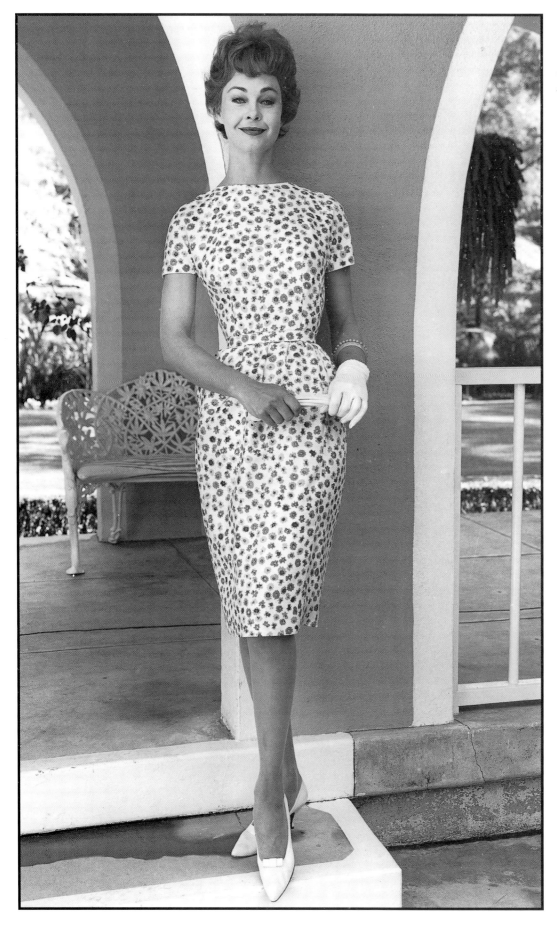

In the late 1950s Lanz was prized for its wash 'n wear daytime dresses. *Courtesy, Jimmy Mitchell.*

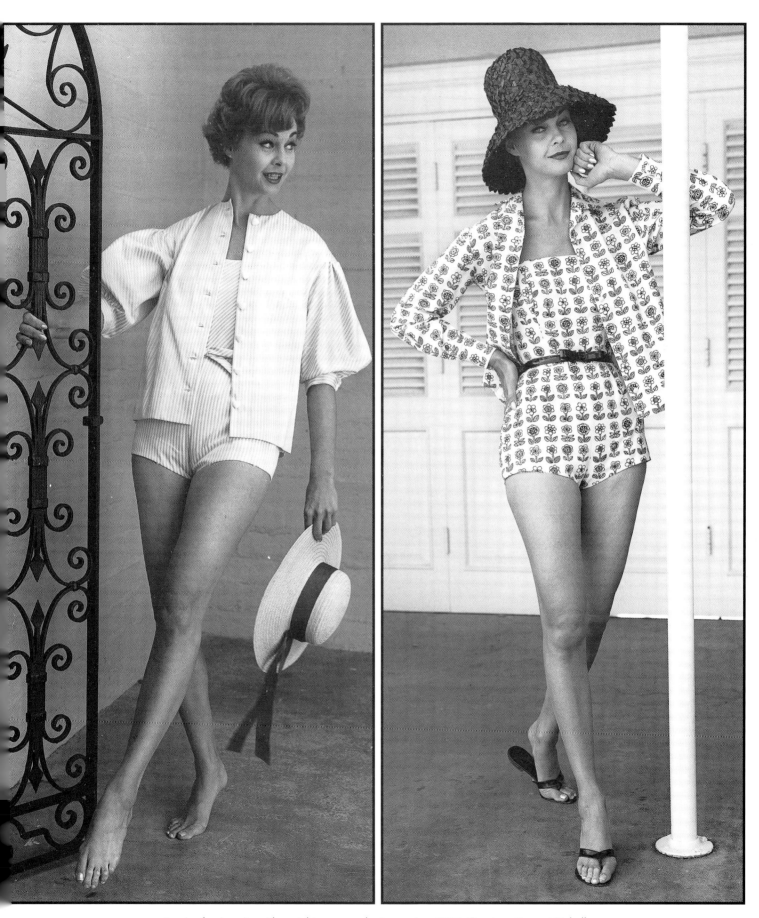

A pair of swimsuits with matching covers by Lanz, circa 1960. *Courtesy, Jimmy Mitchell.*

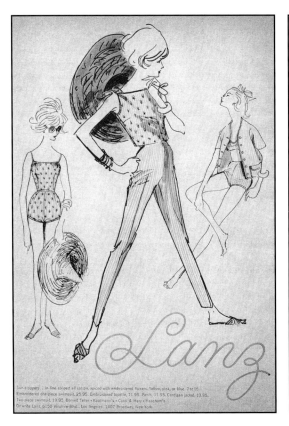

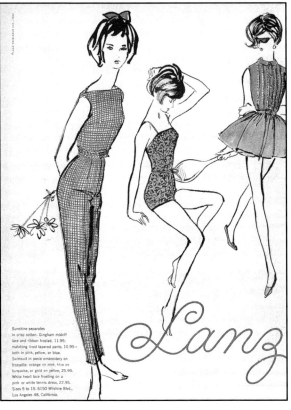

You could build your summer wardrobe around these "sunshine separates" from Lanz, as advertised in April 1962.

Sun-stoppers... in fine striped all cotton, spiced with embroidered flowers. Yellow, pink, or blue. 7 to 16. Embroidered one-piece swimsuit, 25.95. Embroidered topette, 11.95. Pant, 11.95. Cardigan jacket, 13.95. Two-piece swimsuit, 19.95. Bonwit Teller • Kaufmann's • Carol & Mary • Meacham's Or write Lanz, 6150 Wilshire Blvd., Los Angeles; 1407 Broadway, New York.

Sunshine separates in crisp cotton. Gingham midriff lace and ribbon frosted, 11.96; matching lined tapered pants, 10.95— both in pink, yellow, or blue. Swimsuit in posie embroidery on frossette; orange on pink, blue on turquoise, or gold on yellow, 25.95. White heart lace frosting on a pink or white tennis dress, 22.95. Sizes 5 to 15. 6150 Wilshire Blvd., Los Angeles 48, California.

Front and aft views of a shipshape sundress from the early 1960s. For versatility, the middy top could be unbuttoned from the skirt. Value: $35-55. *Author's collection.*

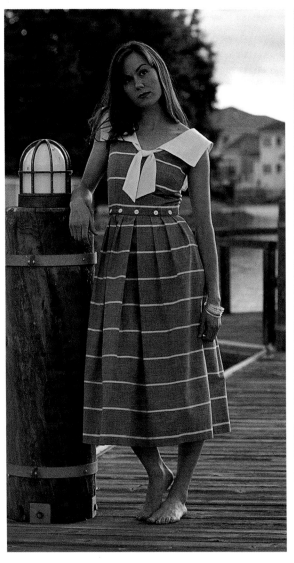

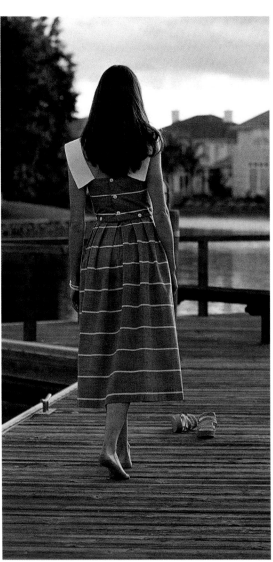

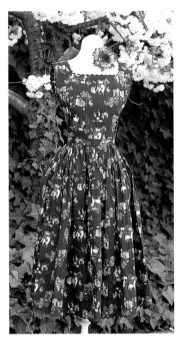

A sundress by Lanz in a "Spirit of '76" print, presumably from the bicentennial year.

For early spring in the late 1960s, a maxi-length jumper in celadon pinwale corduroy with a white eyelet mock petticoat. Attributed to Denise Lanz, for Denise Designs. Value: $25-45. *Author's collection.*

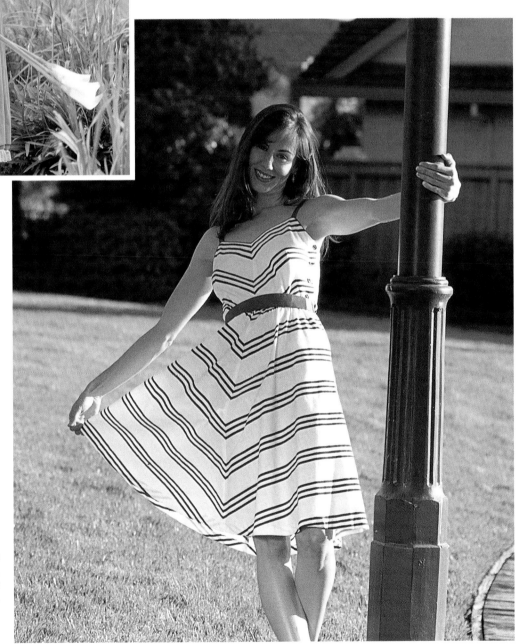

A sweet sundress from the mid-1960s, on Naomi Duffy. Value: $15-25. *Author's collection.*

Patio Party

This sampler of outstanding California labels shows the variety of styles that were marketed as pool 'n patio wear. Many vintage collectors now eagerly seek these casual styles for the fresh charm of their design.

Miss Elliette

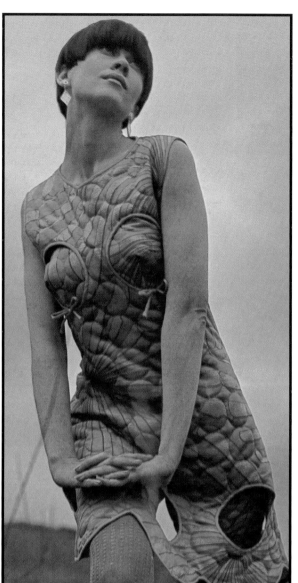

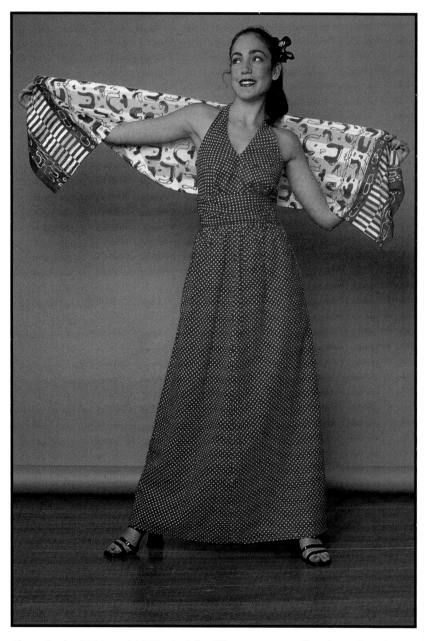

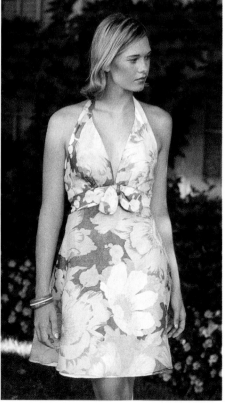

Above: In the 1960s and 1970s, the Miss Elliette company offered pert date dresses like this red-and-white polka dot voile. Value: $55-75. *Courtesy, Cherry.*

Top right: Miss Elliette went futuristic in 1967 with this cotton shift of quilted lime and turquoise.

Bottom right: A daytime date dress in tropical voile, as made by Miss Elliette and worn by Miss Elizabeth Haskett. Value: $35-55. *Courtesy, Cheap Thrills.*

Alex Colman

A darling Capri pant set by Alex Colman, with exotic vest and ball fringe, from 1952. *Courtesy, Jimmy Mitchell.*

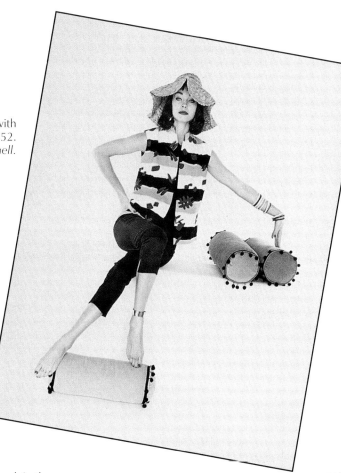

Alex Colman went streamlined and Sanforized, in the Seventies.

The "Alex Colman Closet" campaign gave a fun peek at entire clothing groups, as seen in this ad from the Fall of 1969.

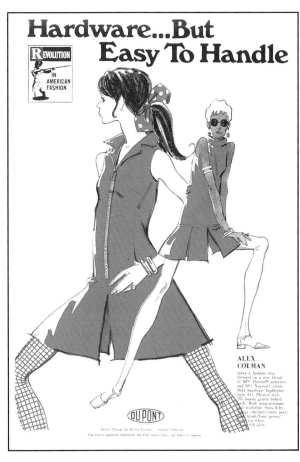

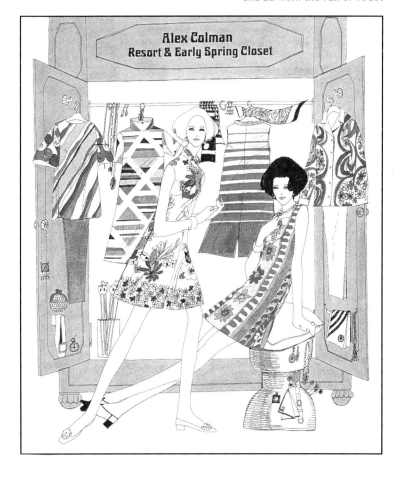

Such a darling fish-scale print (no label, circa 1945). It makes easy-going separates just right for the beach. Value: $125-150. *Courtesy, Lottie Ballou.*

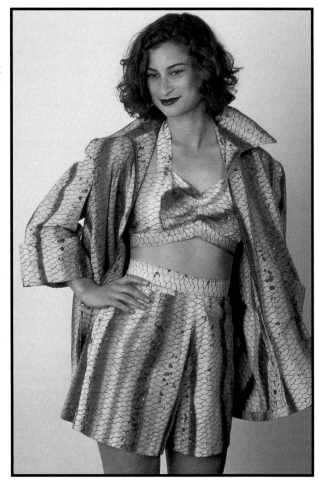

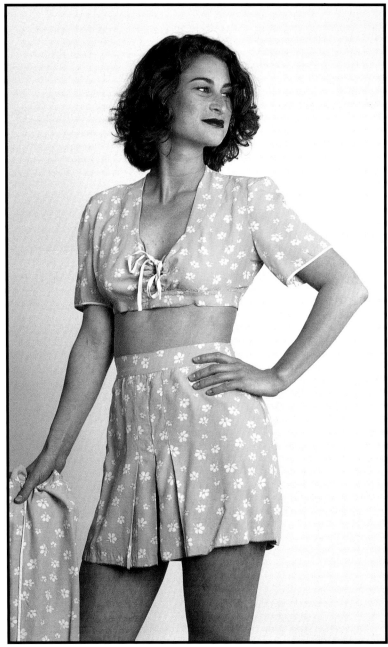

A crop top and shorts in a lemon and white rayon-blend (no label, circa 1938). The set came with a coordinated button-front skirt. Value: $95-125. *Courtesy, Lottie Ballou.*

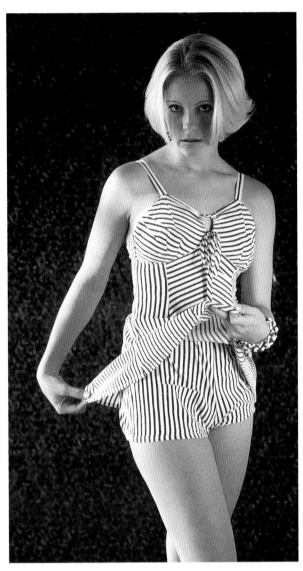

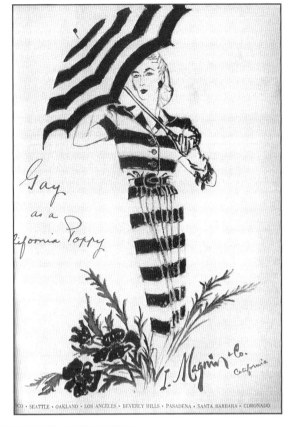

Red was always a popular color for resort. This 1948 ad was designed to lure readers into I. Magnin & Co. for a sundress "Gay as a California Poppy."

This sassy one-piecer in a candy-striper rayon has the look of separates with attached shorts (no label, circa 1950). Value: $75-95. *Courtesy, Luxe.*

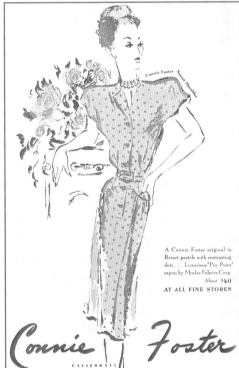

This resortgoer was advertised in December 1945: "A Connie Foster original in Resort pastels with contrasting dots . . . Luxurious 'Pin Point' rayon by Morlee Fabrics Corp. About $40."

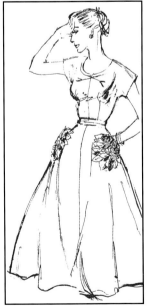

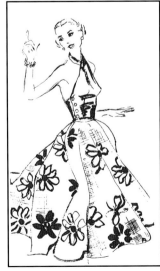

Nathali Nicoli showed linen separates in pale lavender with violet appliqués for pockets. Alex Colman paired a cotton skirt strewn with flowers and a sateen halter top. Both, as featured in *Vogue* on January 1, 1951.

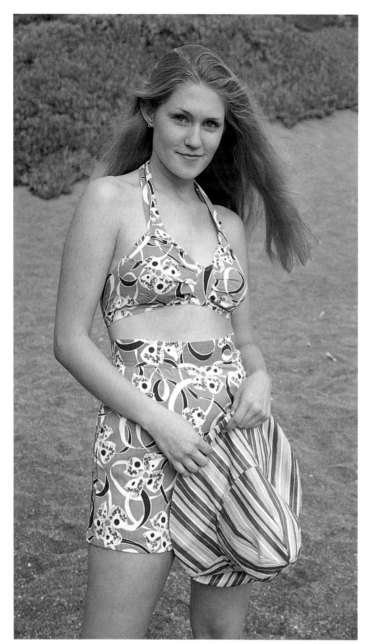

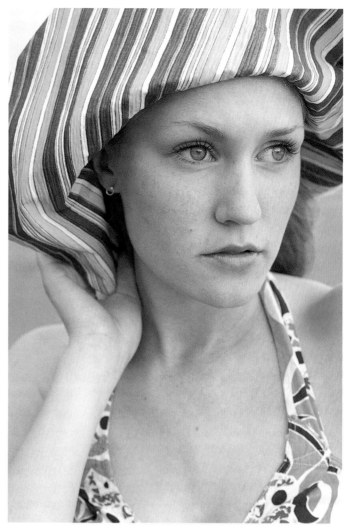

A modern take on the classic sou'wester.

For summers at the shore circa 1940, a halter-top short set in abstract floral cotton (no label). Value: $55-75. *Courtesy, Luxe.*

Two little rompers. At left, an abstract cotton bandeau and skirt (home-made, circa 1950). At right, a skirted suit with shirred back, circa 1955. Value each: $45-55. *Courtesy both, Luxe.*

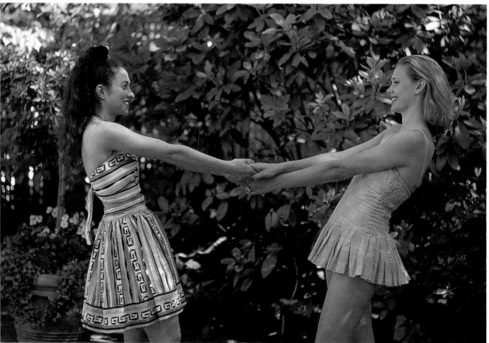

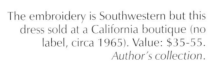

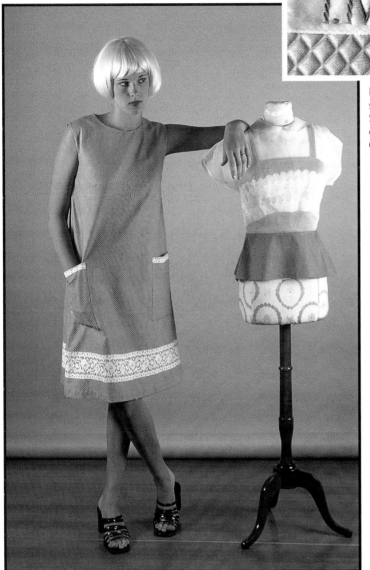

Pink waffle pique and a froth of lace make a sweet skimmer (I. Magnin label, circa 1970). Shown with a party blouse in peach pique overlaid by rayon organza (no label, circa 1960). *Courtesy, Cheap Thrills.*

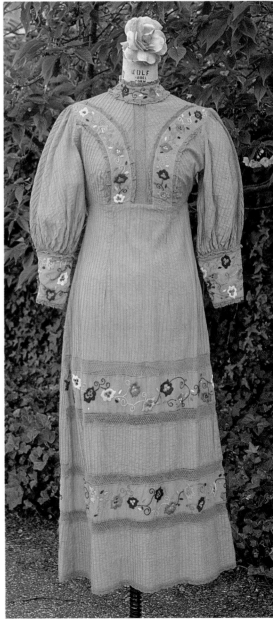

The embroidery is Southwestern but this dress sold at a California boutique (no label, circa 1965). Value: $35-55. *Author's collection.*

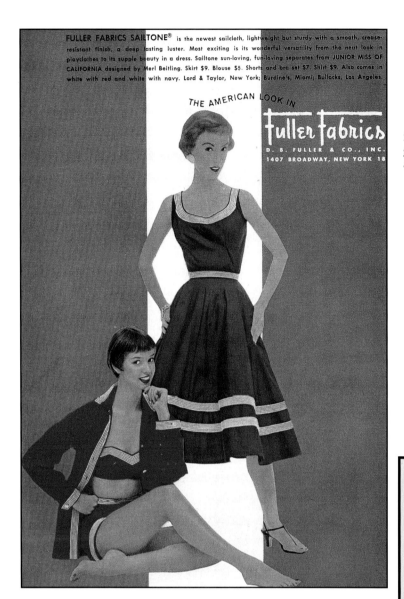

FULLER FABRICS SAILTONE® is the newest sailcloth, lightweight but sturdy with a smooth, crease-resistant finish, a deep lasting luster. Most exciting is its wonderful versatility from the neat look in playclothes to its supple beauty in a dress. Sailtone sun-loving, fun-loving separates from JUNIOR MISS OF CALIFORNIA designed by Merl Beitling. Skirt $9. Blouse $5. Shorts and bra set $7. Shirt $9. Also comes in white with red and white with navy. Lord & Taylor, New York; Burdine's, Miami; Bullocks, Los Angeles.

THE AMERICAN LOOK IN

Fuller Fabrics

D. B. FULLER & CO., INC.
1407 BROADWAY, NEW YORK 18

Sunny separates from the sailcloth group by Junior Miss of California, as advertised in January 1954.

Sailcloth in red *Sailtone* by Fuller Fabrics, trimmed with white yarn. Value: $45-65. *Courtesy, Cheap Thrills.*

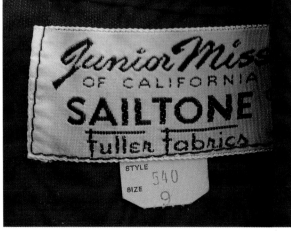

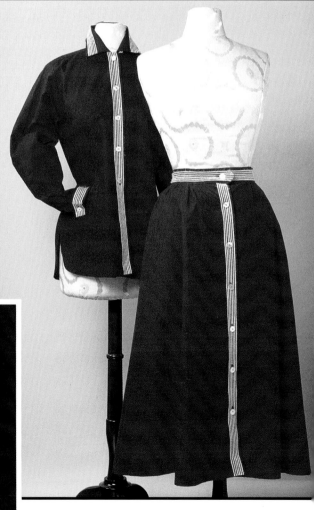

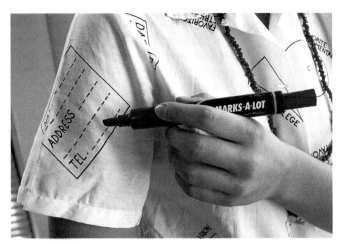

Just put your name and address here!

Autograph hounds loved this set from the late 1950s—perfect for a teen pajama party. In new/old stock with not a *mark* on it (no label). Value: $75-95. *Courtesy, Luxe.*

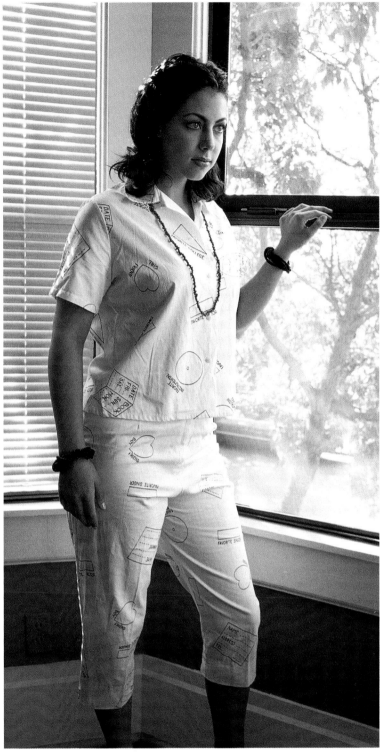

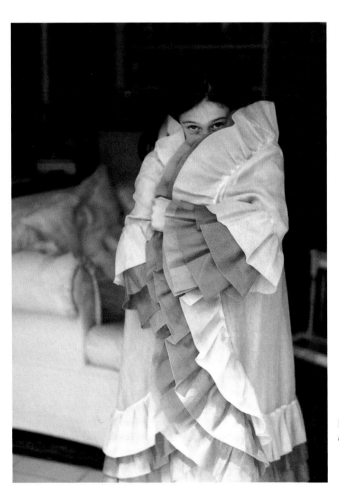

Play dress-up in a ruffled bedjacket, like little Becky Stern (Jos. Magnin label, circa 1980). Value: $25-35. *Author's collection.*

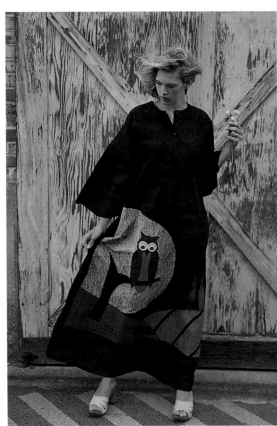

The owl motif is a wise caftan choice for hostess wear, circa 1970. This smart bird is a machine-stitched pastiche of patterns, all in cotton. Label: Ava's Boutique. Value: $25-45. *Author's collection.*

A Juliet dress in lavender rayon with embroidered ribbon trim (no label, circa 1965); it's all about romance for Elizabeth Haskett. Value: $25-45. *Author's collection.*

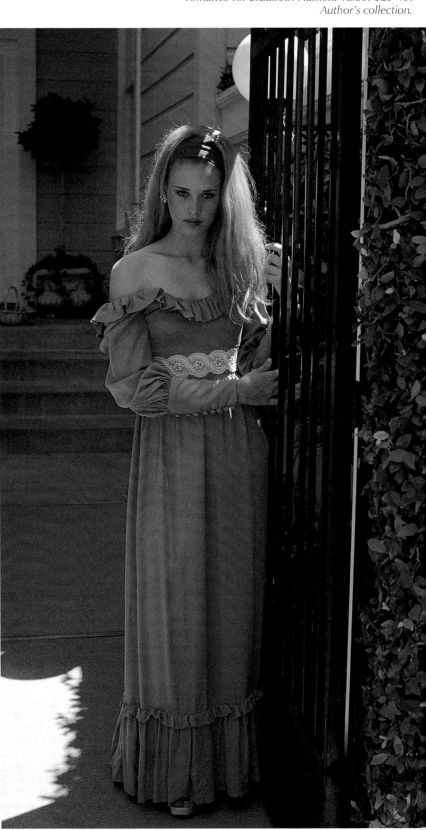

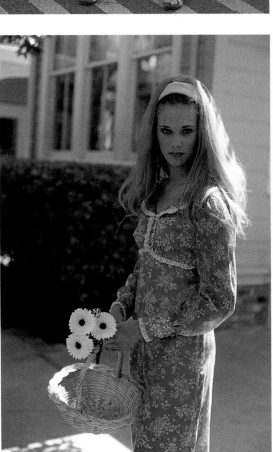

Wildflower posies dot a sky-blue cotton voile gown. Very Hootenanny or hippy chick. By Roberta of California, circa 1965. Value: $15-25. *Author's collection.*

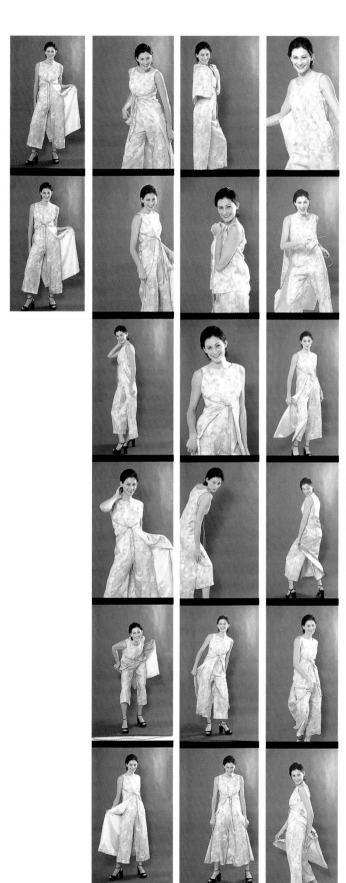

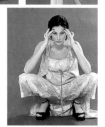

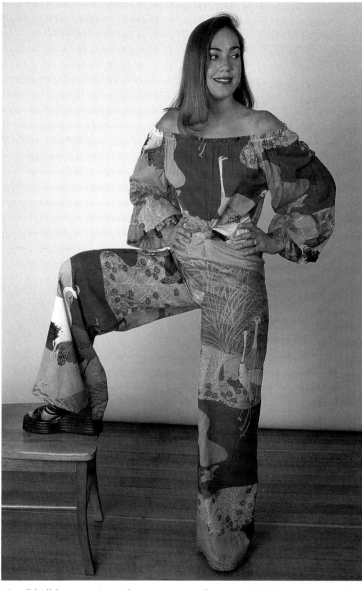

Swell bell-bottoms in a vibrant cotton voile, circa 1970. By Hanae Mori, the high-end designer from California with Pacific Rim sensibilities. Value: $75-95. *Author's collection.*

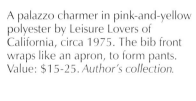

A palazzo charmer in pink-and-yellow polyester by Leisure Lovers of California, circa 1975. The bib front wraps like an apron, to form pants. Value: $15-25. *Author's collection.*

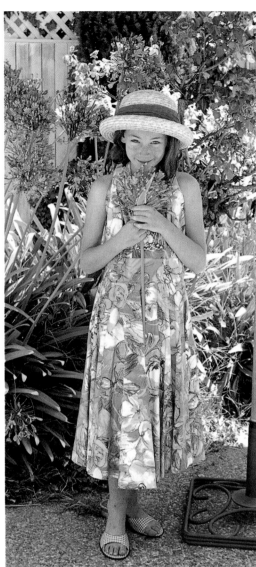

Naomi Stern stops to smell the flowers. She's playing in a sunny print dress by Jan Sue of California, circa 1965. Value: $15-25. *Author's collection.*

Citrus colors pack a punch when mixed with the iridescence of Thai silk, as in this striped patiogoer (Macy's label, circa 1970). Value: $35-55. *Author's collection.*

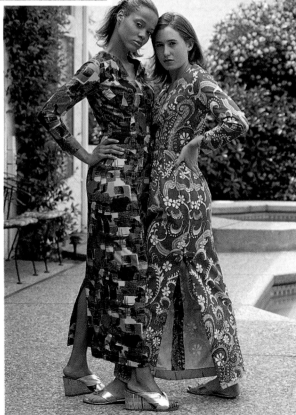

An eye-popping pair in neon-bright polyester (no labels) on Kim and Vesha. In the Sixties, these dresses partied on the best patios. Value each: $25-35. *Author's collection.*

All in the Fabric

There's a strong and symbiotic relationship between the design and manufacture of casual clothing and advancements in fabric technology. For example, the staying power of Lastex and Spandex gave structure to the American swimwear scene. Likewise, the sprightly textiles from California breathed life into sportswear design.

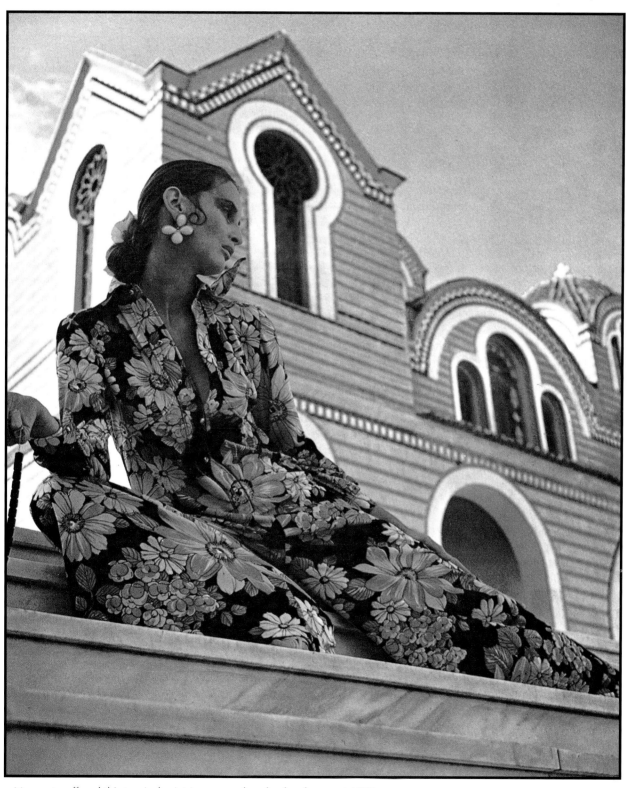

Monsanto offered this tropical print in neon-colored nylon for resort 1970.

A manufacturing region's geography and topography influences the type of textile and clothing designs that will be produced there. From the cult of California, there came about a design *oeuvre* as mixed as an omelet. Take a bit of Hollywood starlet, a pinch of farmer's daughter, a dash of surfer girl, and stir. For spice, add the charm of old Mexico and the exotic allure of traditional Hawaii.

Indigenous Mexican design motifs have inspired craftsmen for generations, from silver jewelers in Taxco to ceramic artisans in Puerto Vallarta. In the 1940s and 1950s, leisure-loving Americans bought all manner of clothing, accessories, and jewelry imbued with fiesta and folkloric motifs. A close look at the Shop Hound mail-order section in vintage *Vogue* magazines will reveal the range of these products, from silver bracelets to huarache sandals.

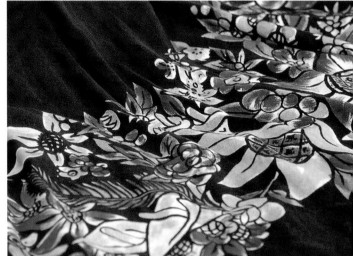

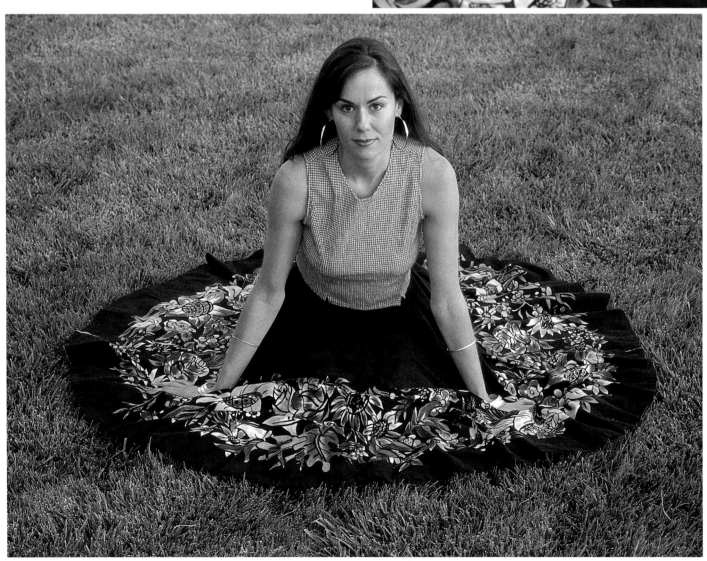

A hand-painted circle skirt from Mexico, one of many ethnic motifs that influenced California textile design.

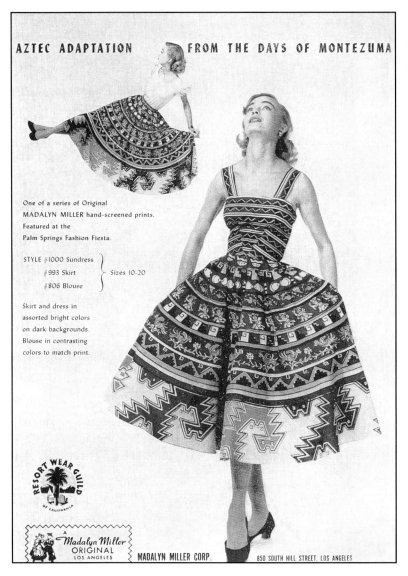

The Resort Wear Guild of California promoted Madalyn Miller at the Palm Springs Fashion Fiesta trade show in 1951. She cut this skirt and sundress from a hand-screened cotton, Aztec motif.

Jamie Saunders plays the saucy senorita in a separates set (no label, circa 1955). Value: Special. *Author's collection*.

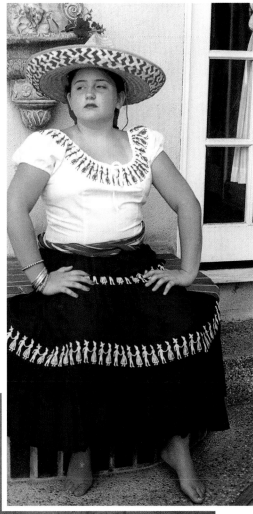

The rows of dancers are machine stitched on cotton.

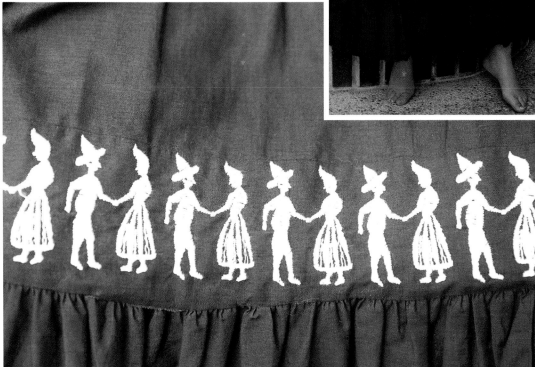

Hawaii has been a popular resort playground for Californians since the 1920s. It's only natural that the relaxed island style would infuse California's design sensibility. From sarong sundress to muu-muus and surfer jams, there are abundant examples of vintage clothing cut from textiles splashed with tropical color. Orchids, ferns, and angel fish frolic on polished cotton and rough barkcloth like a vivid vision of paradise.

The compelling island imagery did not escape the attention of California's garment industry. The *California Stylist* trade journal regularly sponsored joint trade shows and printed a Hawaii themed issue each summer.

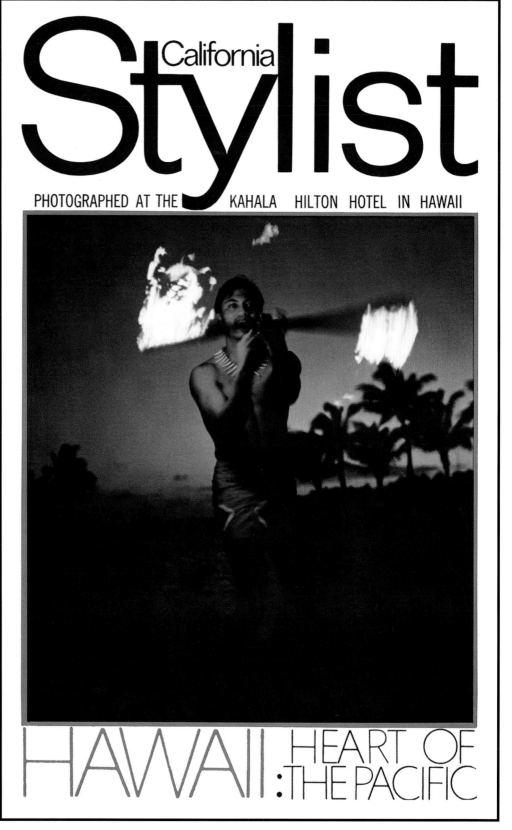

California
Stylist
PHOTOGRAPHED AT THE   KAHALA   HILTON   HOTEL   IN   HAWAII

HAWAII :HEART OF THE PACIFIC

The *California Stylist* featured regular Hawaii issues in the 1960s and 1970s.

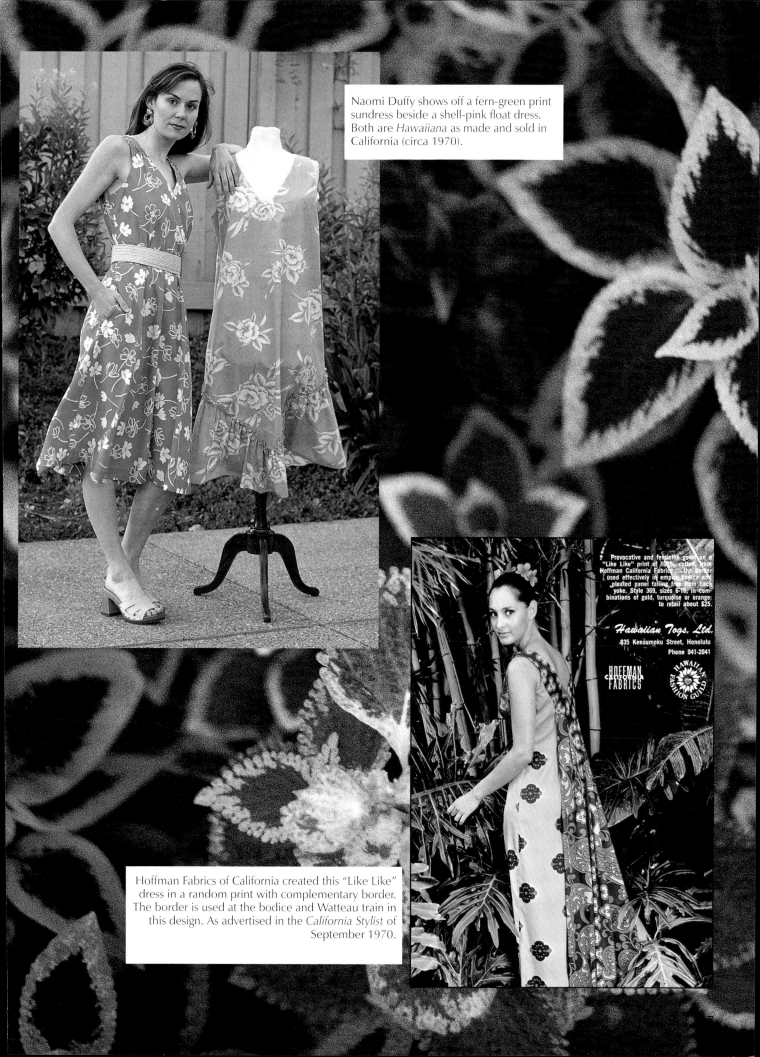

Naomi Duffy shows off a fern-green print sundress beside a shell-pink float dress. Both are *Hawaiiana* as made and sold in California (circa 1970).

Hoffman Fabrics of California created this "Like Like" dress in a random print with complementary border. The border is used at the bodice and Watteau train in this design. As advertised in the *California Stylist* of September 1970.

Provocative and feminine gown on a "Like Like" print of 100% cotton, from Hoffman California Fabrics — the border used effectively in empire bodice and pleated panel falling free from back yoke. Style 369, sizes 6-16, in combinations of gold, turquoise or orange; to retail about $25.

Hawaiian Togs, Ltd.
835 Keeaumoku Street, Honolulu
Phone 941-2041

HOFFMAN
CALIFORNIA
FABRICS

HAWAIIAN
FASHION GUILD

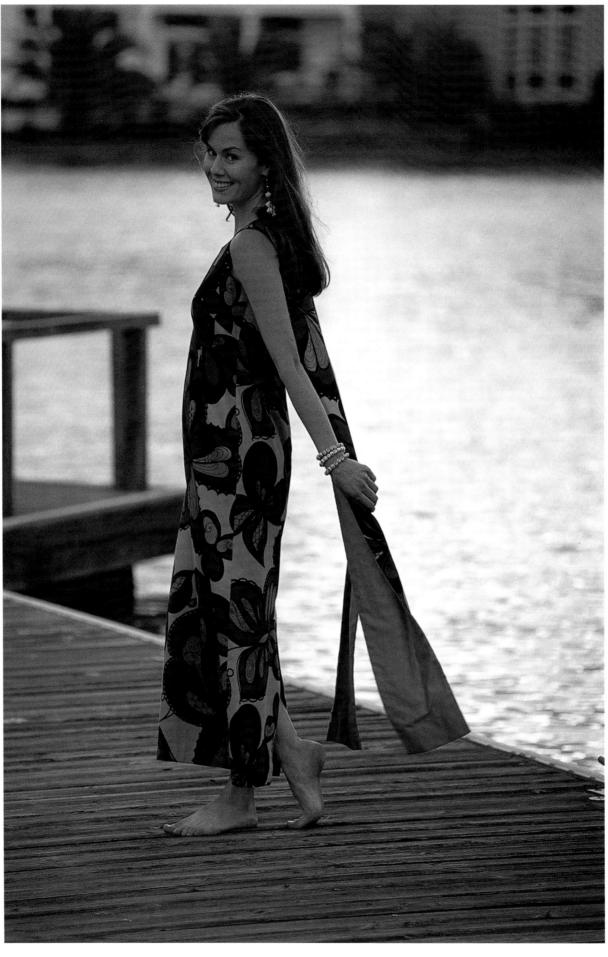

This design with Watteau train, similar to the "Like Like" dress on previous page, is grandly casual in a hostess gown by Lauhaha of Hawaii. It's in a barkcloth surrealist print in tones as deep and cool as the Pacific Ocean.

chapter 4

DENIM REVELATIONS

"Denim. Jeans. America is a country that prides itself on its toughness, individuality, and youthful spirit; it is difficult to find a common thread woven through time that has remained unchanged and as popular or durable as jeans made of cotton denim."
— David Little, *Vintage Denim*, 1996.

The easy popularity of blue jeans lies in their durability and comfort. In turn, those characteristics result from using the right fabric and method of construction, and tailoring a garment to its specific task. It's all about performance, and it's the same principle that drove the development of specialty fibers and fabrics for sportswear.

The story of how denim was first imported to America is apocryphal. In it is embodied the very heart and soul of a young and nearly class-free nation, a melting pot population intent on bettering itself through hard work and ingenuity. It's the story of Levi Strauss, a young immigrant from Bavaria who sought his fortune in the gold fields of California.

On January 24, 1848, gold was discovered by a carpenter at the Sutter sawmill on the outskirts of what is now Sacramento. Word spread like wildfire once the assay content was confirmed, and the great Gold Rush was on, attracting every dreamer and get-rich-quick hopeful from the East Coast and Europe.

In 1850, it attracted the twenty-year-old Strauss, who hoped to sell canvas to the miners for tents and wagon covers. He soon found that customer demand was for sturdy work clothes that could stand up to the physical abuse of panning, picking, and scrabbling for gold.

After consulting with a tailor, the enterprising Strauss began making "waist-high overalls" from his supply of canvas tent. When that ran out he turned to a durable, diagonal-weave cotton known as *serge de Nimes* (so called after the region in southern France where it had been the stuff of peasant dress for generations).

Strauss imported it by the boatload, in trading ships manned primarily by Genoese sailors. (The word "denim" comes from *de Nimes*, and "jeans" from Genoese.) Denim can be dyed in many colors but Strauss preferred indigo, a deep blue dye imported from India. Thus, the cloth of blue jeans culture was born. Now, for the cut.

Denim fabric derives from the *de Nimes* region of France. This example from the mid-1800s bears a striking similarity to the "peasant dress" style worn by young Americans in the mid-1900s.

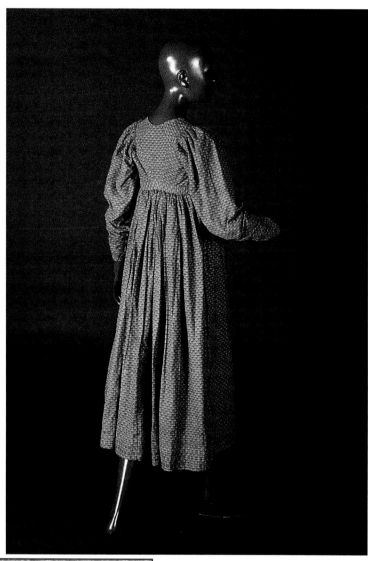

Workers at the Levi Strauss plant in the early 1900s. *Courtesy, Levi Strauss & Co. Archives*.

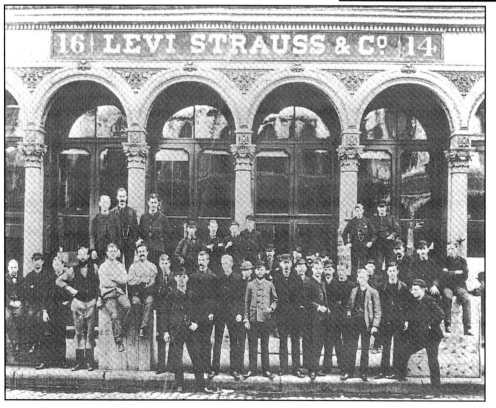

The overalls that Strauss churned out were the sturdiest on the market, but they were still not strong enough to withstand wear-and-tear by hard-working prospectors. In 1873, after more discussions with local tailors, Strauss conceived the idea of fastening seams and pockets with rust-proof copper rivets. He even riveted the fly-front crotch, until a miner got too close to the campfire, and realized the heat-conducting properties of copper!

Before patenting his copper-rivet design in May 1873, Strauss added a trademark double-arc of stitching on the back pockets to suggest an American eagle's outspread wings. Also, the crotch rivet was dropped. In 1886, Strauss placed a leather patch at the waistband to commemorate an advertising stunt whereby two horses failed in the attempt to tear apart a pair of his jeans. That was it; the classic Levi's style is essentially the same today.

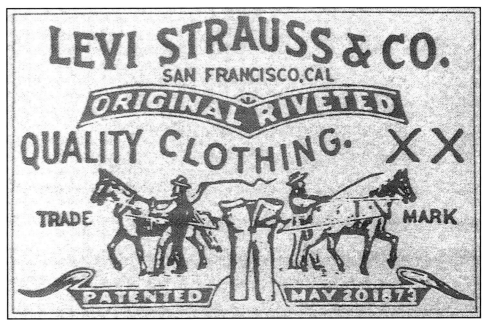

The commemorative leather patch. *Courtesy, Levi Strauss & Co. Archives.*

By the 1900s, the digs were panned out and the gold rush was over, but the demand for jeans was stronger than ever. Farmers, cowhands, and lumberjacks universally wore jeans, buying them from catalogs and hardware stores. When the dustbowl forced sharecroppers into a westward migration they arrived in California clad in blue jean overalls. As Iain Finlayson wrote in his erudite book *Denim*: "No money, no status, no hope beyond basic survival. Denim is still redolent of the mythic hardship of the Great Depression, of tenacity in adversity, of the human spirit that endures even in despair."

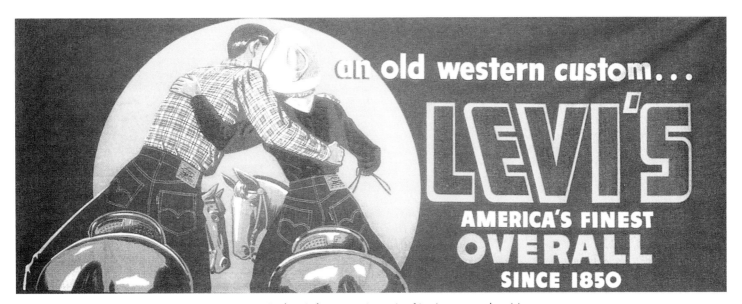

Romance was in the air for a courting pair of Levis, on an advertising banner from the 1950s. *Courtesy, Levi Strauss & Co. Archives.*

Blue denim took on different mythic qualities thanks to the Golden Era of Hollywood. Along with historical epics and screwball comedies, Hollywood peddled the romantic Wild West in the persona of singing cowboys like Gene Autry, Tex Ritter, and Roy Rogers.

Blue jeans were also the staple of dude ranch dressing, a trend that swept the country in the 1940s and 1950s. At once wholesome and sexy, denim was soon being seen on everyone from pinup girls to the girl-next-door. Billed "a family tradition" by eager advertisers, jeans became standard attire for after-school and weekends, as worn by the postwar generation.

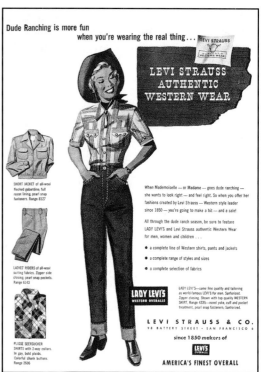

Levi Strauss introduced its *Lady Levi's* line in the 1940s. This ad from Spring 1951 was geared to "the dude ranch season."

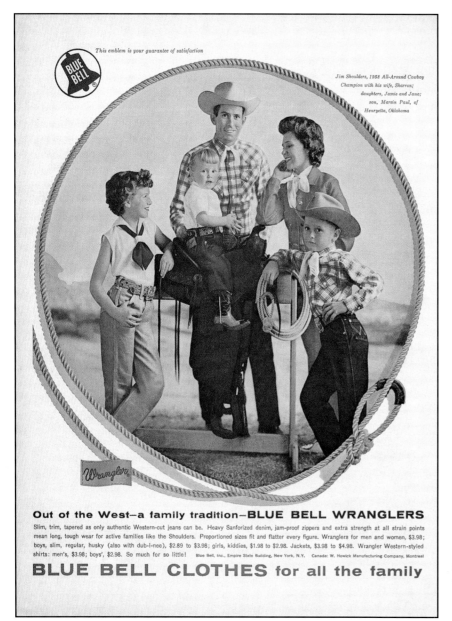

In 1958, Blue Bell (a New York based competitor of Levi's) advertised Wrangler jeans as a family tradition. They are shown worn by the All-Around Cowboy Champion Jim Shoulders and family.

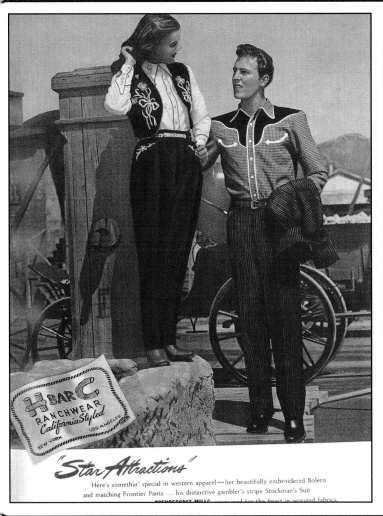

An essay on the craze for western clothing in the *California Stylist* of January 1951 declared blue jeans a clothing tribute to the "easier, freer" way of life out West.

"We understand the vogue of dude ranches has transformed the American resort picture. Also, we find the western influence rampant in our finest residential sections. Successful young executives, space-minded and freedom-loving men from all walks of life . . . have in the backs of their thoughts a little spot of land where they can raise garden truck and flowers, stable their own horses, live an untrammeled life far from the confusion of the city."

Duded up in H-BAR-C Ranchwear that was "California Styled." As advertised in 1948, these duds were not denim, but woolen worsted.

"Star Attractions"

Here's somethin' special in western apparel — her beautifully embroidered Bolero and matching Frontier Pants . . . his distinctive gambler's stripe Stockman's Suit.

It was only natural that denim should transition into a fashion statement as Americans refined the concept of sports dressing. In April 1951, *Vogue* ran an article on denim with an emphasis on classic good looks. "Riddle: what is the summer equivalent of grey flannel, that tailors firmly, holds its shape, washes as easily as your own hands, combines with braid or dotted Swiss or embroidery or with jewels, is cut for the city and pared for the beaches, and dyed and woven a dozen new ways? Denim it is, of course."

"Diamonds and Denims are a Girl's Best Friends." Royal Fabrics and Junior House teamed up in this 1951 advertisement for rhinestone-studded beachwear.

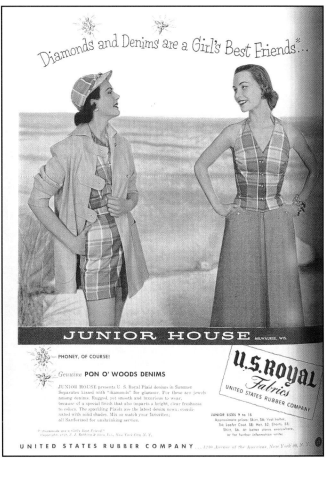

*Diamonds and Denims are a Girl's Best Friends**...

JUNIOR HOUSE MILWAUKEE, WIS.

PHONEY, OF COURSE!

Genuine PON O' WOODS DENIMS

U.S. ROYAL Fabrics
UNITED STATES RUBBER COMPANY

UNITED STATES RUBBER COMPANY

*V*ogue had its editorial finger on the pulse of denim's versatility, one factor that would make the fabric a wardrobe staple for many years: "On these pages, we've briefed the denim outline for summer, from jeans to bathing suit to traveling costume. But there's even more to denim than that. There are denim coats, denim dusters. There are denim's new colourings . . . There is denim's texture . . . There are new details . . . And finally, there is the fact of denim's opacity, which means . . . you can wear denim over nothing, nothing at all."

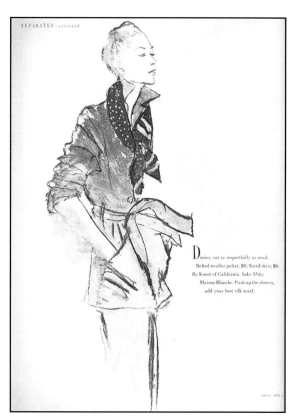

Denim, cut as respectfully as wool.
Belted stroller jacket, $8; flared skirt, $6.
By Koret of California. Saks 34th;
Maison Blanche. Push up the sleeves,
add your best silk scarf.

There's more to denim in a belted stroller jacket and slim skirt. This is a 1949 design by Koret of California.

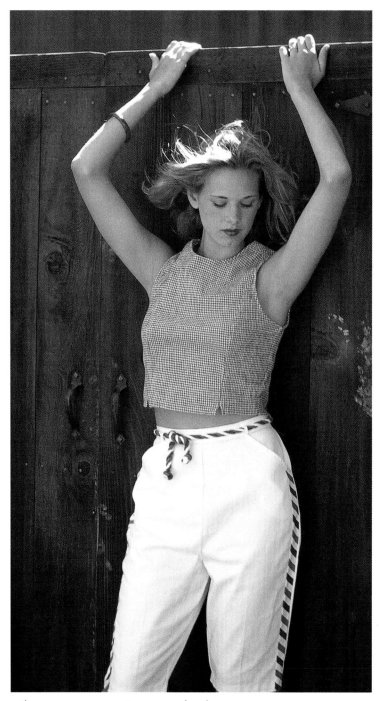

Then as now, summertime meant freedom to dress in denim or "nothing at all."

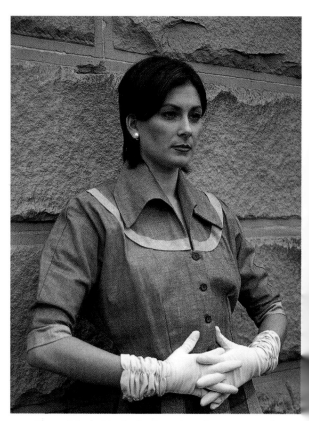

The suit jacket is denim in a clean brown, one of the new colorings.

174

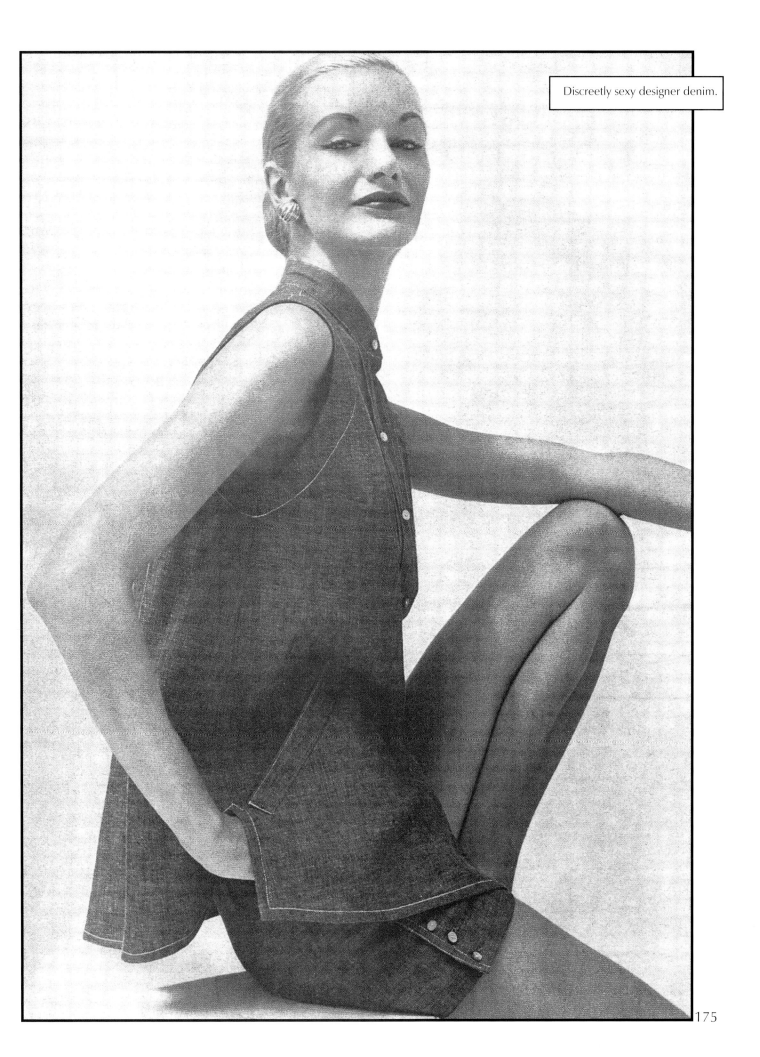

Discreetly sexy designer denim.

175

By the 1960s, denim had evolved from the utilitarian stamp of working-class clothes into an icon of carefree youth. The tan leather Levis 501 label was like a badge of honor on the backsides of college war protesters in the 1960s. Denim—so red, white and blueable—soon became a background for patches of torn American flags and other fabric graffiti of the Vietnam war protesters. It wasn't long before the garment industry had standardized the flag motif, making it a less incendiary emblem of youthful fashion.

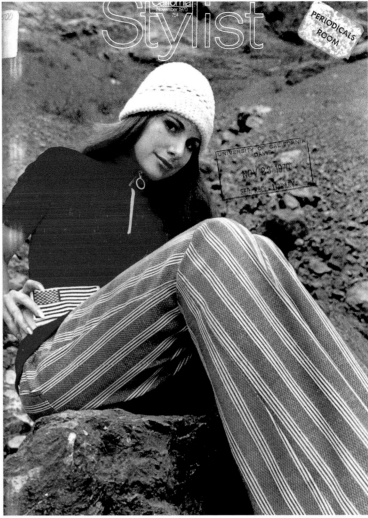

The flag motif went from war protest to fashion statement, as seen on this cover from the November 1970 issue of the *California Stylist.*

Peter Max, who captured pop culture in art posters of the 1960s, also dabbled in designing printed denim. This 1971 ad from Jump Suits Ltd. of Dallas spoke of giving Max "carte blanche to go ahead and do the spaciest designs he could think of."

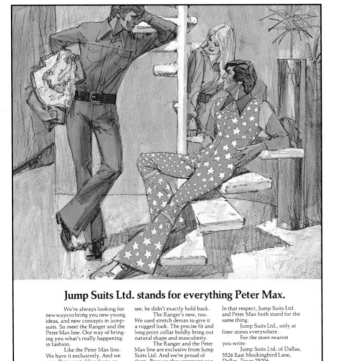

It was all a far cry from days gone by, when the same Levis 501 label had been worn by farmers and factory workers. Now it was street-wise stuff, as Finlayson explained eloquently: "It was, so far as possible, classless and anonymous, consciously and deliberately symbolic of revolution that did not require clothes to symbolize position in a social hierarchy."

Ironically, but predictably, the working class did not want to remain anonymous. In dress, the under-privileged aspired to symbols of status and wealth, and favored jeans that were embellished with studs, fringe, and embroidery. The *frisson* of 1970s socio-political struggles was manifested, on the fashion front, in the form of *customized* denim.

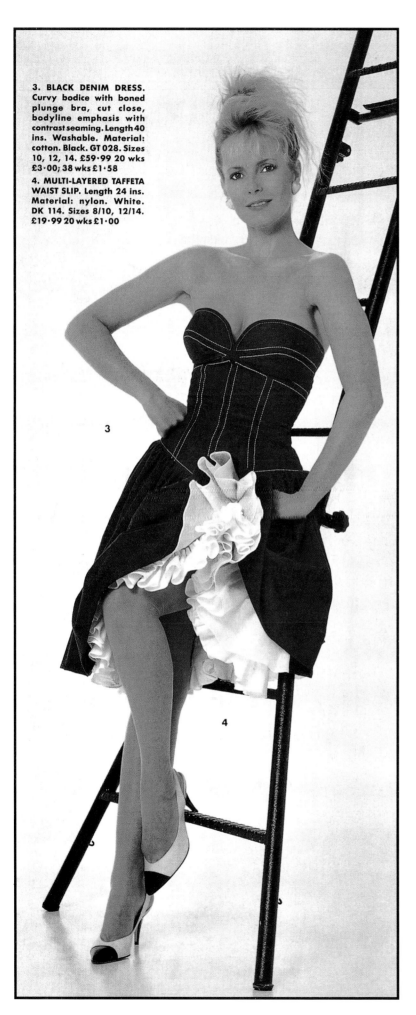

3. **BLACK DENIM DRESS.**
Curvy bodice with boned plunge bra, cut close, bodyline emphasis with contrast seaming. Length 40 ins. Washable. Material: cotton. Black. GT 028. Sizes 10, 12, 14. £59·99 20 wks £3·00; 38 wks £1·58

4. **MULTI-LAYERED TAFFETA WAIST SLIP.** Length 24 ins. Material: nylon. White. DK 114. Sizes 8/10, 12/14. £19·99 20 wks £1·00

3

4

Rock stars like Jim Morrison and Janis Joplin wore jeans on stage and off, advancing its radical chic image. In New York and Paris, couturiers realized they were losing *haute* chick customers to the counterculture of denim at the counter of any major department store. Designer denim came of age in the 1980s; soon, nothing but the price tag came between a *fashionista* and her Calvins.

Within recent memory, denim evolved again into a new kind of un-uniform. This time, it was for the class of corporate elite who introduced the "Casual Friday" ethic into the workplace. First it was confined to computer rich Silicon Valley, but the lure of denim was strong. By now, Casual Friday has become a fashion cult in the glass-and-steel towers of corporate America. White-collar workers are outfitted in blue denim, fitting tribute to the enduring quality of this hard-working fabric.

A sexy, flirty look in black denim over white eyelet. As modeled by Cheryl Ladd in 1986, for William Travilla's Dallas-inspired catalog line.

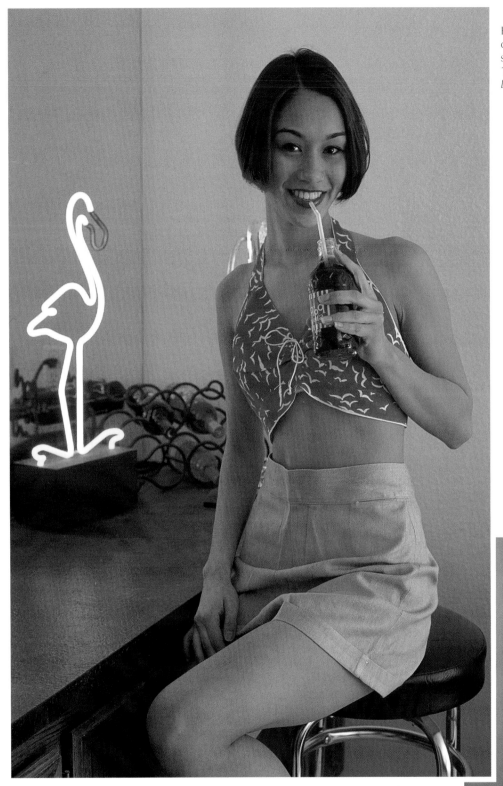

Kristi Talbert enjoys a soda in her smart car-hop denim shorts and cotton seabreeze halter (both no label, circa 1950). Value, each: $15-25. *Courtesy, Luxe.*

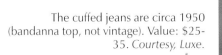

The cuffed jeans are circa 1950 (bandanna top, not vintage). Value: $25-35. *Courtesy, Luxe.*

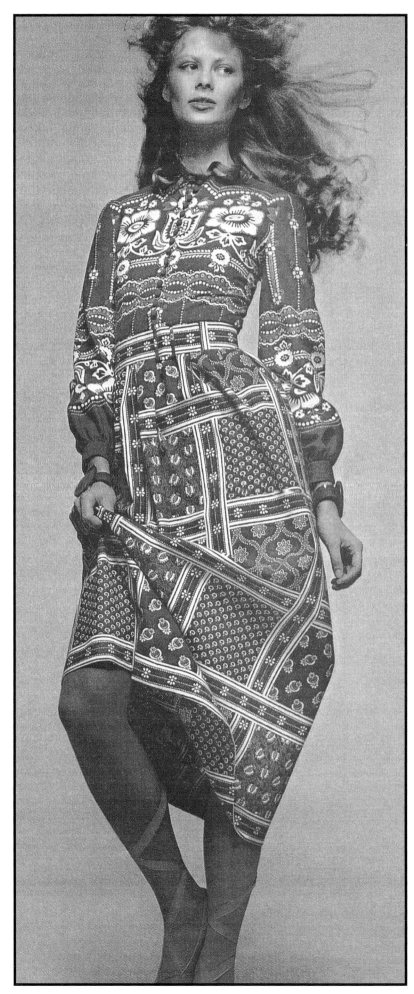

Oscar de la Renta was one of many European designers who used denim in the 1970s. This gown mixes the Western heritage of blue denim and bandannas.

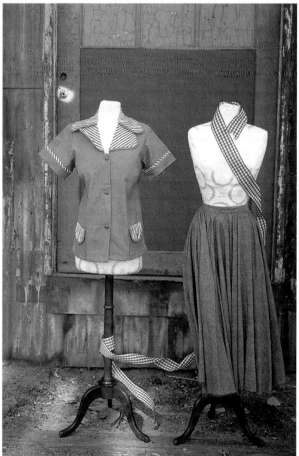

The jacket lapels arc in a black-and-white awning stripe (no label, circa 1945). Shown with a circle of black denim trimmed in red rickrack (no label, circa 1955). Value each: $15-25. *Courtesy both, Cheap Thrills.*

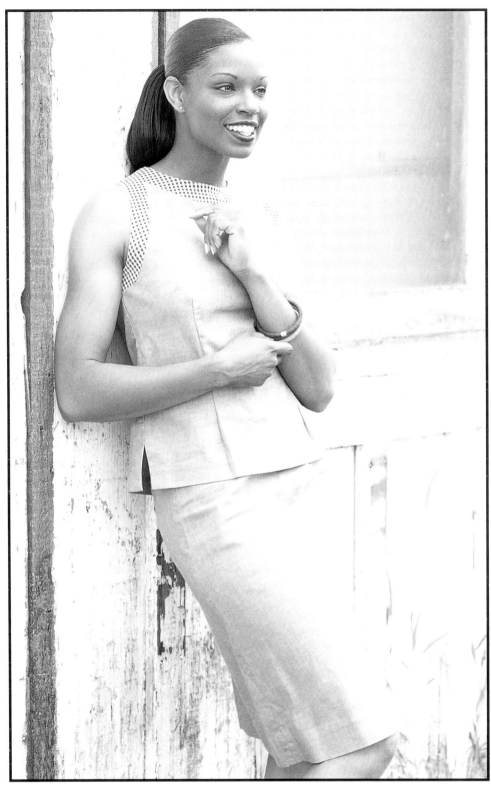

On Regina Williams, a cute two-piece dress in whitewashed blue denim with red-and-white gingham (no label, circa 1965). Value: $15-35. *Author's collection.*

For everyday wear, circa 1965. The red stitching repeats the gingham facing. From the aptly-named label "Country Looks by Bobbie Brooks." Value: $15-25. *Courtesy, It's About Time.*

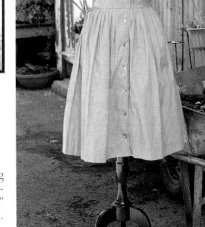

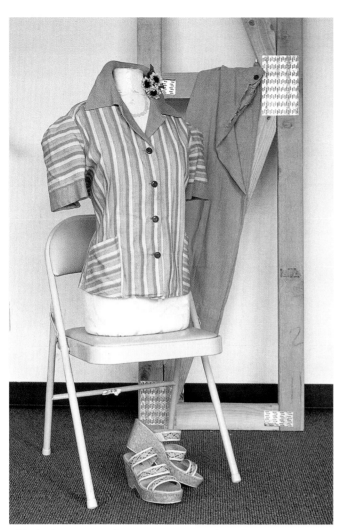

This denim pant set shows great 1940s style. Value:
$75-95. *Courtesy, Luxe*.

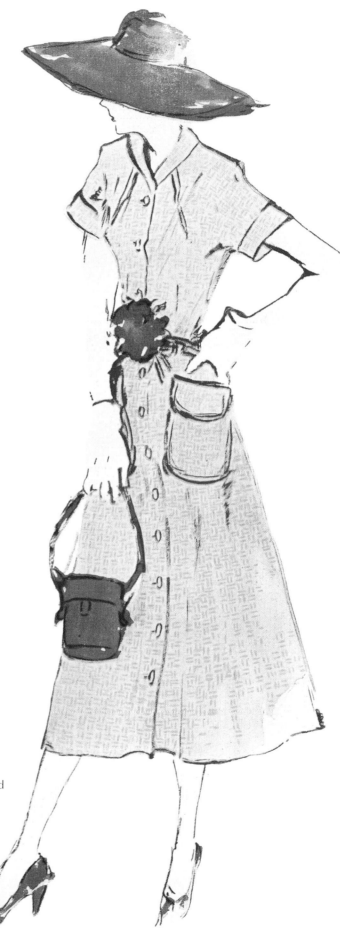

A summer cooler in blue chambray sparked
with red, as shown in May 1950.

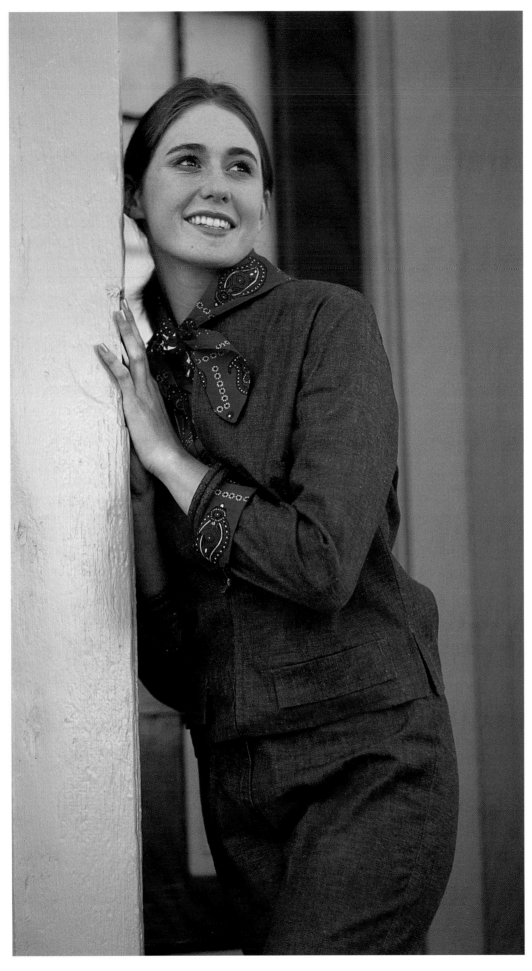

A three-piece denim slack set with Western style. The jacket is lined in red bandanna print, matched to a sleeveless blouse with attached kerchief in lieu of a collar. By Ardee of California, circa 1965. Value: $75-95. *Courtesy, The Way We Wore.*

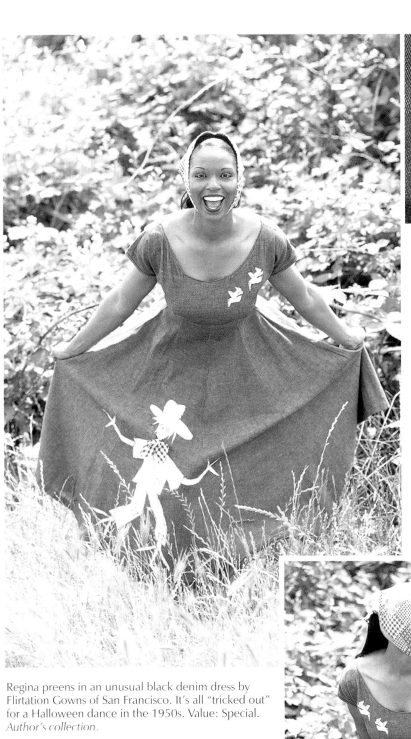

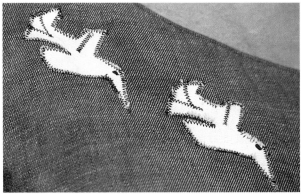

The gingham insets are of a scarecrow, crows, and haystack.

Regina preens in an unusual black denim dress by Flirtation Gowns of San Francisco. It's all "tricked out" for a Halloween dance in the 1950s. Value: Special. *Author's collection.*

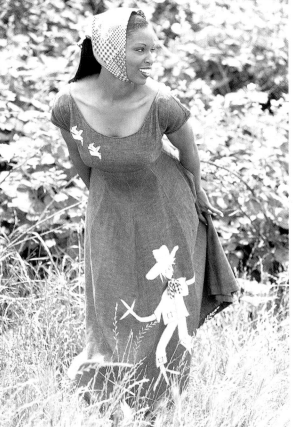

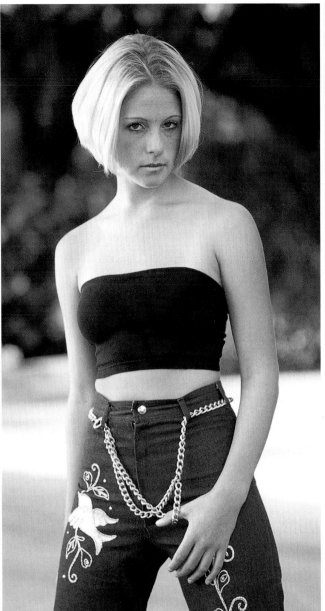

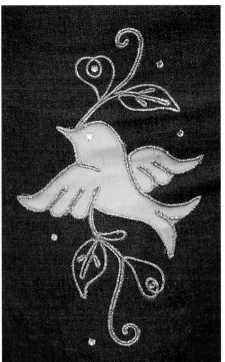

The bird in a gilded cage is flying free.

A good example of glitzed-up designer denim (no label, circa 1980). Value: Special. *Courtesy, Cheap Thrills.*

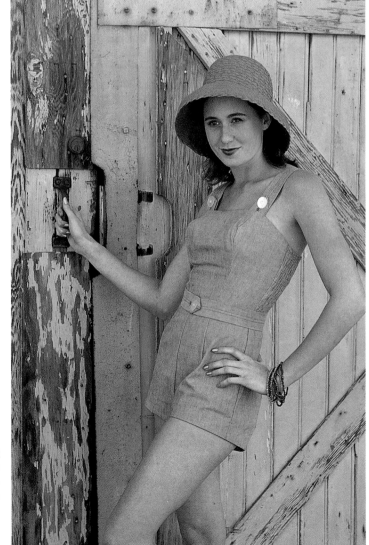

Pink denim forms a cute boy-short swimsuit on Kim Davidson. By John Weitz of California, circa 1965 (see also p. 8). Value: $25-35. *Courtesy, Cheap Thrills.*

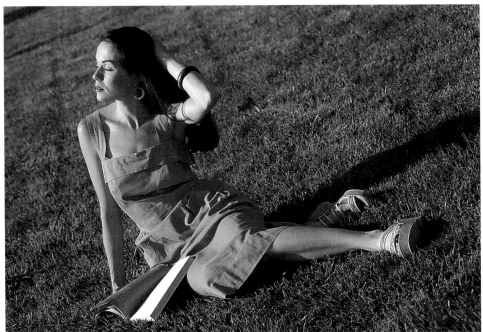

Naomi Duffy lounges in a sundress in pink chambray, close cousin to denim, circa 1955 (no label). $35-55. *Author's collection.*

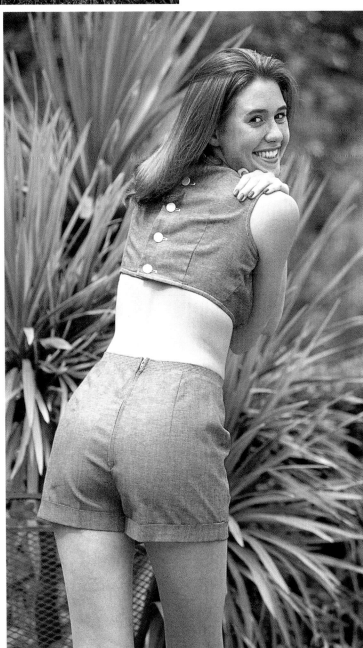

Kim's all buttoned-up in a pink denim play set by Koret, circa 1960. Value: $55-75. *Courtesy, The Way We Wore.*

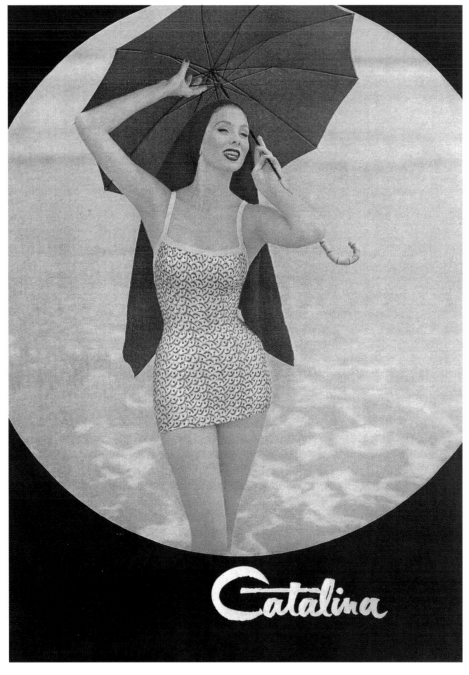

A bread-and-butter style, from Catalina's 1956 line. It's the type of style that invokes fond memories of Fifties fun.

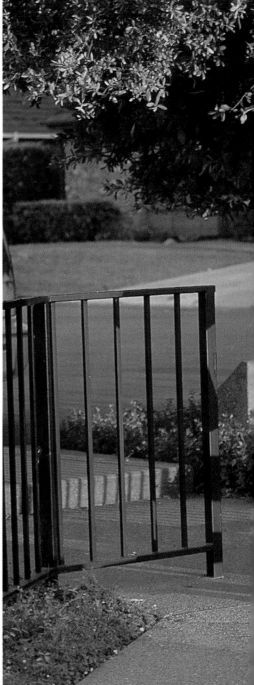

Sportswear is a complex business, built on fabric innovations as well as style. This simple tennis dress is a case in point, featuring wash 'n wear machine embroidery.

Many of the photos in this book include a price range or "value" which represents what the garment would cost in the vintage clothing marketplace, exclusive of auction. Readers should be aware that vintage clothing varies widely in price depending on the type of market (estate sale vs. dealer) and proximity to the region of original manufacture. Of course, as with any collectible, vintage clothing is priced according to condition, rarity, and age.

For purposes of the price ranges shown in this book, readers should assume that the garments are in good, if not mint condition. That said, bear in mind that few collectibles elicit such a strong personal reaction. With the exception of museum curators and designers, many collectors intend to *wear* the garments—not just display them. Thus, size directly affects value. The most darling swimsuit in a sample size may be less costly than a flawed one in a wearable size.

So what's the bottom line on valuation? Just that vintage clothing is priced by supply and demand, with an emotional escalation factor. And yet, there's a bonus to be found by reason of that same emotional factor, in wearing a truly unique garment or in preserving something that represents an important period in fashion history.

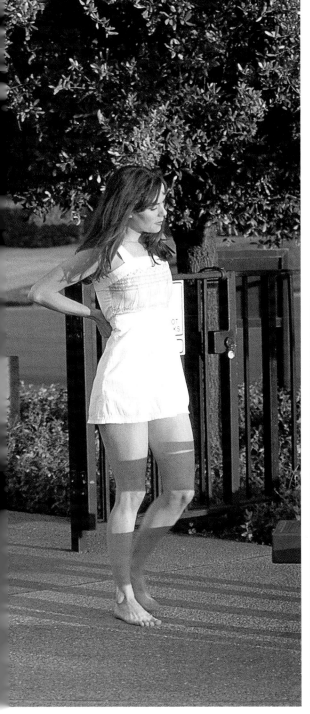

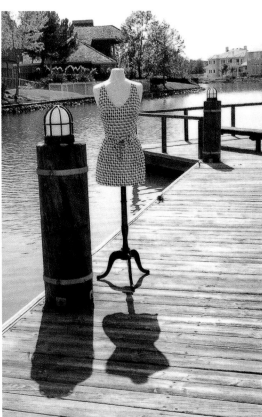

Every company that had a jazzy, sexy line would also offer conservative styles. For example, this discreetly skirted swimsuit is by Cole of California (circa 1955), the company that built its name on Hollywood glamour. Value: $15-25. *Author's collection.*

DEALER DIRECTORY

Cheap Thrills
1217 21st Street
Sacramento, CA 95814
(916) 446-1366
Contact: Marlene Davenport

Cherry
185 Orchard Street
New York, NY 10002
(212) 358-7131
Contact: Cesar Padilla

It's About Time
2104 "J" Street
Sacramento, CA 94814
(916) 446-5944

Lottie Ballou
130 West "E" Street
Benecia, CA 94510
(707) 747-9433
Contact: Margo Adams

Luxe
2453 Lombard Street #104
San Francisco, CA
(415) 468-7482
Contact: Lis Normoyle

The Way We Wore
1094 Revere Way (A-29)
San Francisco, CA
(415) 822-1800
Contact: Doris Raymond

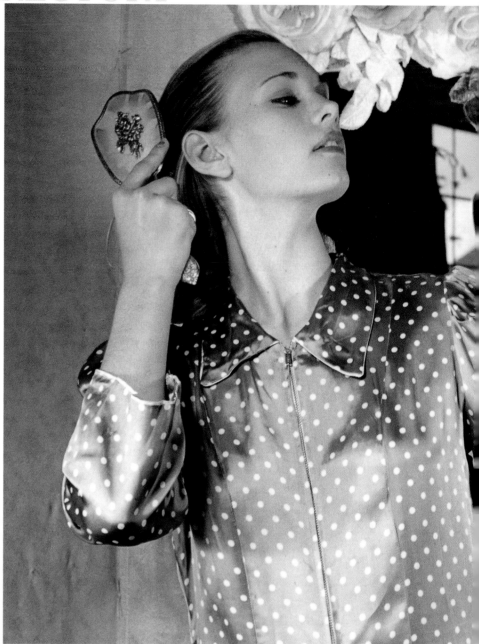

Look backward to the legacy of California design. This polka-dot rayon sateen dressing gown is by Mode O'Day (circa 1940). Value: $35-45. *Courtesy, It's About Time.*

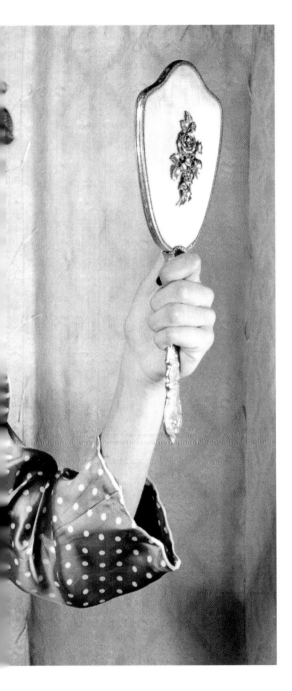

Appliqué: The process of stitching a fabric motif onto a fabric background; usually, the fabrics contrast.

Bandeau: An elasticized, strapless bra or bodice cut straight across the top.

Bateau: A neckline that runs from shoulder to shoulder, with a shallow curve.

Bikini: An abbreviated two-piece swimsuit with a bra top and triangle panties cut below the navel. The name derives from the Bikini Atoll site of early Atom-bomb testing.

Bloomer: A style of swimsuit bottom that is loosely gathered at the leg by elastic banding. The name derives from loose undergarments worn by women in the 1800s, which were proposed as a model for streetwear by the dress reformist Amelia Bloomer.

Blouson: A style of swimsuit top that is bloused just below the natural waistline.

Boy-cut: A style of swimsuit bottom cut long and slim, like a schoolboy's shorts.

Cap: A short sleeve that just covers the top of the arm, sometimes incorporated into vintage swimwear and cover-ups.

Dotted Swiss: Sheer, almost transparent cotton flecked with white dots.

Gabardine: Firm twilled cotton or wool, with diagonal ribbing on the right side.

Gingham: A yarn-dyed plain woven fabric made into stripes, checks and plaids. Usually cotton, but may be silk or rayon. Usually, one color is contrasted with white, but it may be contrasted with black.

Halter: A style of swimsuit top fastened by a strap or ties at the back of the neck, leaving the back and shoulders bare.

HyMo: Trade name for the interfacing of good quality that was used by many vintage manufacturers.

Jacquard loom: A semi-automatic loom on which various fabrics (cotton, satin, velvet) may be woven into elaborate patterns with a system of "punch cards." Invented by Joseph-Marie Jacquard in the mid-1800s, and still in use today for brocades and damasks.

Jams: Knee-length swim trunks, popularized by surfers.

Jersey: A plain, machine-knit fabric, originally a woolen manufactured in the nineteenth century on the English Channel island of Jersey, for use in fishermen's clothing.

Lastex: The trademark name for the elastic yarn made by U.S. Rubber (aka Royal) Fabrics, by wrapping strands of natural fiber around a rubber core; developed in the 1930s.

Maillot: A one-piece swimsuit style, close-fitting with a scoop back, sensible enough for athletic swimming (pronounced may-oh).

Panel: A style of swimsuit bottom that stretches across the lower front hips, simulating a skirt, in the front only; popularized by Catalina for the first Miss America Beauty Pageant.

Peplum: Flounce of fabric extending from waist to hip; typically the lower part of a suit jacket, but may be inset at the waistline of a dress. Popular in the 1940s and early 1950s.

Piqué: Crisp cotton with a honeycomb weave, often used for cuffs and collars.

Rayon: Man-made fabric from a glucose base of plant fiber, with good draping and dying qualities. A less expensive version (viscose rayon) may be made from a glucose base of wood pulp, but it does not handle as well.

Rhinestones: Faux diamonds, cut from glass or crystal. Generally clear with silver foil backing, although they may be tinted in pastel or iridescent shades with gold backing.

Silk: Originally from China, silk was brought to Europe in the twelfth century as a luxury fabric. Soft and shiny, silk drapes easily and dyes well. Depending on the weave, silk may be dense or sheer in weight.

Soutache: Braid or yarn stitched down to form a design.

Spandex: An elasticized, artificial fiber composed mainly of segmented polyurethane; a refinement of Lastex, it was introduced in the 1950s.

Thai: A type of silk, woven with iridescent luster.

Topless: The name given by Rudi Gernreich to his black knit swimsuit with a panty bottom, and no top but for a V-shaped set of suspenders; introduced in 1964.

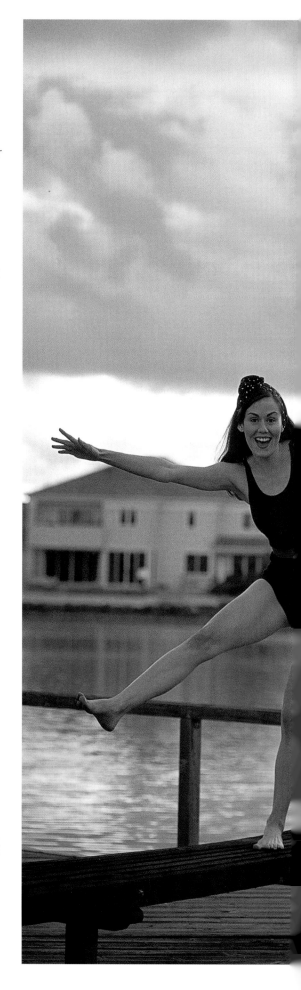

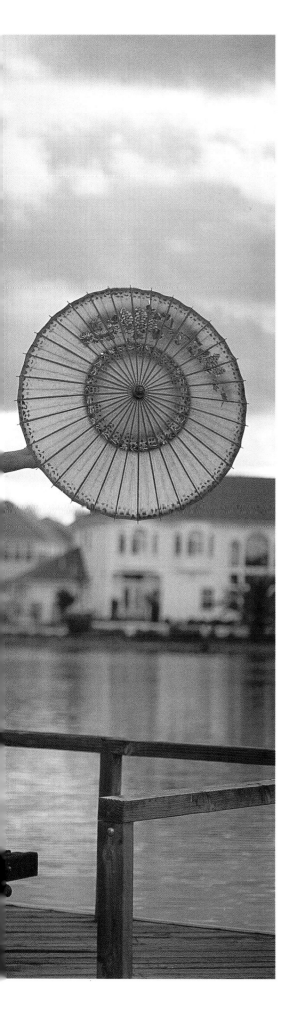

Thong: The bottom part of a Unisex suit cut to expose the cheeks; introduced by Gernreich in 1984; may be worn topless.

Velvet: Double-woven silk, cotton, or rayon with a short, thick pile. Very plush and soft to the touch.

Velveteen: A form of velvet in single-woven cotton or rayon; less plush and soft than velvet.

Voile: Veil; French. A fine, sheer, lightweight fabric generally woven from natural fiber (silk or cotton).

Watteau: The sixteenth century artist whose portraits of ladies from the French court often showed them in robes with a long, loose train hanging not from the waist but the shoulders; now, the name for a similar train or drape.

Shake it up in a jazz-baby swimsuit with modern spirit.

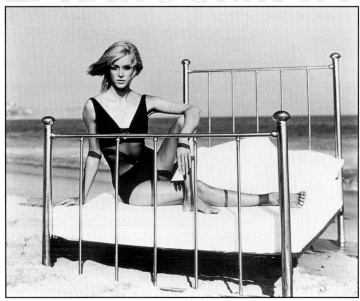

Finlayson, Iain. *Denim*. Norwich, 1NG: Parke Sutton, Ltd., 1990.

Hawes, Elizabeth. *Why A Dress?* New York City: Viking, 1942.

Lencek, Lena and Gideon Bosker. *Making Waves*. San Francisco: Chronicle Books, 1988.

Little, David with Larry Bond. *Vintage Denim*. Salt Lake City: Gibbs-Smith, 1996.

Maeder, Edward. "That California Look; textile designs by Elza of Hollywood." Los Angeles: Los Angeles County Museum of Art, 1986.

Martin, Richard. *American Ingenuity, Sportswear 1930s-1970s*. New York City: Metropolitan Museum of Art, 1995.

Martin, Richard and Harold Koda. *Splash! A History of Swimwear*. New York City: St. James Press, 1995.

McDowell, Colin. *Forties Fashion and The New Look*. London: Bloomsbury Publishers, 1997.

Milbank, Caroline Rennolds. *New York Fashion*. New York: Harry N. Abrams, Inc., 1987.

Reilly, Maureen. *California Couture*. Atglen, Pa: Schiffer Publishing, Ltd., 1998.

Reilly, Maureen. *Interview with Anne Cole*. Commerce, CA: May and July, 2000.

Yohannan, Kohle and Nancy Nolf. *Claire McCardell, Redefining Modernism*. New York: Harry N. Abrams, Inc., 1998.

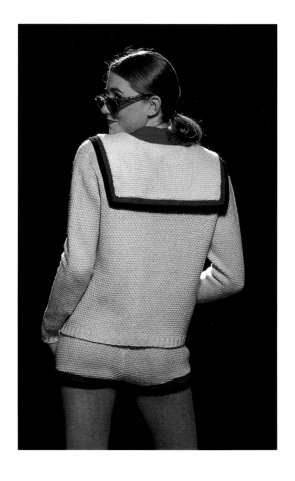

[Note: Some books are out-of print, but are still listed because they may be available through a library or used bookstore.]

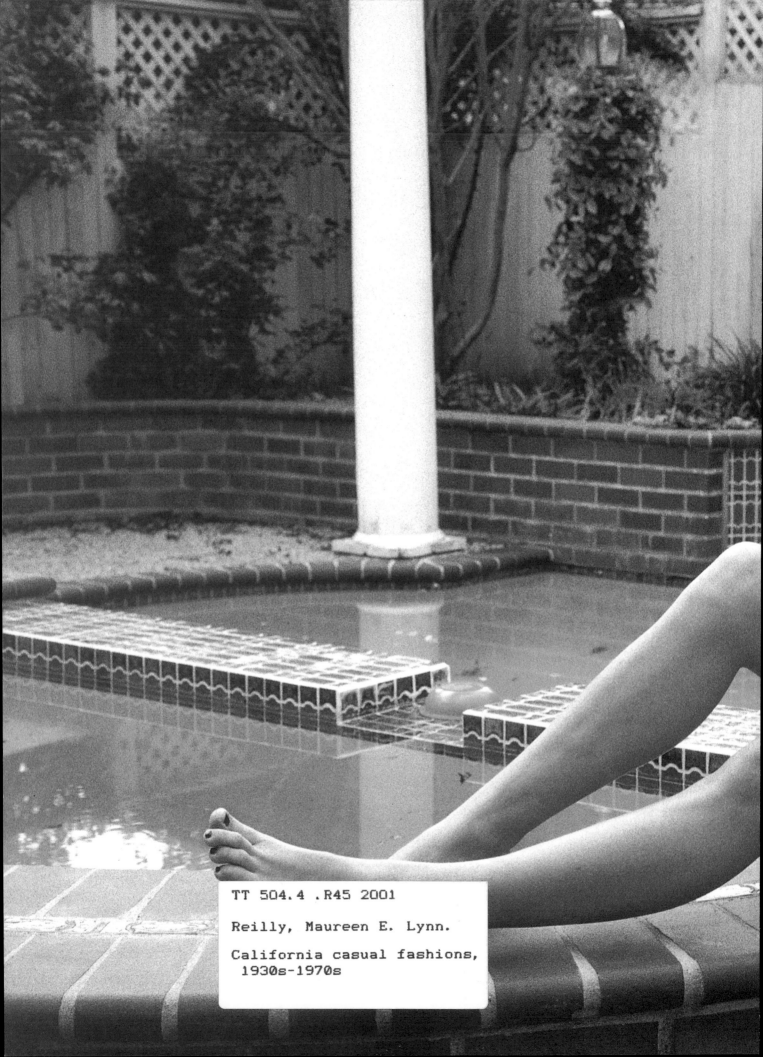